Handbook of Biochemistry for Paramedical Students

for Courses in
Medical Laboratory Technology, Allied Health Sciences and Nursing (As per Competency Based Revised Curriculum for BSc Nursing given by Indian Nursing Council)

Handbook of Biochemistry for Paramedical Students

for Courses in
Medical Laboratory Technology, Allied Health Sciences and Nursing (As per Competency Based Revised Curriculum for BSc Nursing given by Indian Nursing Council)

Anithasri Anbalagan MBBS, MD (Biochemistry), DNB
Senior Assistant Professor
Department of Biochemistry
Government Villupuram Medical College
Villupuram, Tamil Nadu

Suryapriya Rajendran MBBS, MD (Biochemistry)
Professor
Department of Biochemistry
Saveetha Medical College and Hospital
Chennai, Tamil Nadu

CBSPD

CBS Publishers & Distributors Pvt Ltd

New Delhi • Bengaluru • Chennai • Kochi • Kolkata • Lucknow • Mumbai
Gujarat • Hyderabad • Jharkhand • Nagpur • Patna • Pune • Uttarakhand

Handbook of
Biochemistry
for **Paramedical Students**

ISBN: 978-93-5466-819-7

First Edition: 2025

Reprint **2026**

Published by **Satish Kumar Jain** and produced by **Varun Jain** for

CBS Publishers & Distributors Pvt Ltd

4819/XI Prahlad Street, 24 Ansari Road, Daryaganj, New Delhi 110 002, India
Ph: 011-23266838, 23289259 Website: www.cbspd.com
e-mail: delhi@cbspd.com

Corporate Office: 204 FIE, Industrial Area, Patparganj, Delhi 110 092, India
Ph: 011-49344934 Fax: 011-49344935 e-mail: publishing@cbspd.com; publicity@cbspd.com

Branches

- **Bengaluru:** Seema House 2975, 17th Cross, K.R. Road, Banasankari 2nd Stage Bengaluru 560 070, Karnataka, India
  Ph: +91-80-26771678/79 Fax: +91-80-26771680 e-mail: bangalore@cbspd.com
- **Chennai:** 18/8B, Subbarayan Street, Shenoy Nagar, Chennai 600 030, Tamil Nadu, India
  Ph: +91-44-42032115, 45022115 e-mail: chennai@cbspd.com
- **Kochi:** 42/1325, 1326, Power House Road, Opposite KSEB, Power House, Kochi, 682018 Kerala, India
  Ph: +91-484-4059061–65 Fax: +91-484-4059065 e-mail: kochi@cbspd.com
- **Kolkata:** 147, Hind Ceramics Compound, 1st Floor, Nilgunj Road, Belghoria, Kolkata 700056 West Bengal, India
  Ph: +91-33-25633055/56 e-mail: kolkata@cbspd.com
- **Lucknow:** Basement, Khushnuma Complex, 7 Meerabai Marg (behind Jawahwar Bhawan) Lucknow 226001, UP, India
  Ph: +91-522-4000032 e-mail: tiwari.lucknow@cbspd.com
- **Mumbai:** PWD Shed, Gala No. 25/26, Ramchandra Bhatt Marg, Next JJ Hospital, Gate No. 2 Opp. Union Bank of India, Noorbaug Mumbai 400009, Maharashtra, India
  Ph: +91-22-66661880/89 e-mail: mumbai@cbspd.com

Representatives

• **Gujarat** • **Hyderabad** • **Jharkhand** • **Nagpur** • **Patna** • **Pune** • **Uttarakhand**

For trade terms please contact customercare@cbspd.com
For general enquiries please contact info@cbspd.com

Preface

With the showers of blessings from the Almighty we render this humble piece of knowledge to our beloved students who have set in their career journey with us. The young minds of students is filled with eagerness and enthusiasm as they step into the college from their schooling. Biochemistry is the first subject they land up with new molecules and new reactions. To make these molecules friendly to the students and to increase the affinity of the students towards biochemistry we were constantly in search of a suitable way.

The first thing that was striking is to make it appear simple. The very appearance of size and content of the book must encourage the readers to get attached to it. This book is the outcome of such a beginning. Secondly, students enjoy the subject when they understand it easily. Fear and omission of subject is due to the burden of difficult concepts and complex ideas. This book is a solution for this complexity. This is written in such a way, the mother feeds the cooked nutritious meal to the baby. It is readily absorbed and assimilated. This makes biochemistry a tasty subject for the students. Third is the ultimate purpose of the students which is to pass through the subject successfully in their examination. The book is a complete compilation of all the exam-oriented topics and also enables the students to present concisely what they have learnt throughout the entire year and to increase their creativity of presentation.

Every word in the book was written from the shoes of the students so that they cherish and enjoy the subject when they understand and comprehend its contents.

Any kind of constructive criticism and suggestions are welcome that can make this book a best companion of biochemistry for the students.

Anithasri Anbalagan
Suryapriya Rajendran

Acknowledgements

Our sincere gratitude to Prof Poonguzhali Gopinath, Head, Department of Biochemistry, Government Villupuram Medical College, Dr N Ananthi, Professor and Head, Department of Biochemistry, Saveetha Medical College and Hospital and Dr GSR Kedari, Professor, Department of Biochemistry, Saveetha Medical College and Hospital who ignited this lamp of knowledge.

We are thankful to our seniors and colleagues in the Department of Biochemistry. Dr K Tamilmani, Dr G Gunavathi, and Dr C Sathishkumar of Government Villupuram Medical College, Dr S Vinod Babu, Dr Gurupavan Kumar Ganta, Dr Kunjumon Ittira Vadakkan, Dr D Merriwin, Dr V Veena, Dr PJ Padmini, Dr R Hemalathaa, Dr M Sabarinathan, Mr H Ashwin Raj, Mrs E Keerthika and Mr Deepak Rajan of Saveetha Medical College and Hospital, who were a great support in our venture of bringing out this book.

We thank Ms P Kalavathy and Mr G Kapil Dev, Lab technicians of Government Villupuram Medical College and Ms T Ishwarya and Ms D Monisha, Lab technicians of Saveetha Medical College and Hospital for their constant encouragement and assistance.

We thank our teachers and seniors in JIPMER, Puducherry, who sowed the seeds of Biochemistry in us and guided us in acquiring the skills of teaching biochemistry.

Last but not the least, our heartfelt gratitude to our family members who are the internal energy that propel us.

We thank the entire publishing team of CBS Publishers & Distributors especially Mr YN Arjuna Senior Vice President—Publishing, Editorial and Publicity for his guidance and support throughout the publishing process, Mrs Ritu Chawla—GM Production, Mr Dinesh Chandra Arya DTP operator and Mr S Muralidaran Area Sales Manager, Chennai, for bringing out this book successfully. My cordial gratitude to Dr Yashi Bajpai Editional Assistant for her concern and earnest contribution in the making of this book.

Anithasri Anbalagan
Suryapriya Rajendran

Contents

Section III: Practical Biochemistry

Section IV: Clinical Biochemistry

Section V: Metabolism

Section VI: Nutrition

Section VII: Molecular Biology, Immunology

SECTION

I

General Laboratory Principles

1. Laboratory Hazards
2. Laboratory Safety Measures
3. Biomedical Waste Management
4. Glasswares
5. Blood Collection Techniques (Phlebotomy)
6. Anticoagulants and Vacutainers
7. 24 Hours Urine Collection and Urine Preservatives
8. Types of Solutions
9. Buffers and pH Indicators
10. Quality Control
11. Reference Ranges
12. Calibration

CHAPTER

1

Laboratory Hazards

A hazard is anything that may cause injury, harm, or damage. **Laboratory hazards are risks or dangers encountered when performing work in a laboratory.** Despite the widespread belief that laboratories are safe places to work, there is a very high risk of hazards. When handling hazardous materials, people are required to follow specific protocols to protect others as well as themselves. Here are a few examples of common laboratory dangers along with their management strategies.

Classification of laboratory hazards

- Laboratory hazards
  - Physical hazards
    1. Electricity
    2. Fire
    3. Equipment
    4. Glass ware
  - Chemical hazards
    1. Flammable
    2. Corrosive
    3. Toxic
    4. Explosive
    5. Carcinogens
  - Biological hazards
    1. Blood
    2. Culture media
    3. Urine
    4. Stool
    5. Body fluids

Physical hazards: Hazards that occur by physical agents. They include electrical faults, cuts from broken glassware, fire from leaking gas cylinders, etc.

1. **Electricity:** Potential exposures to electrical hazards can result from faulty electrical equipment/instrumentation or wiring, damaged receptacles and connectors, or unsafe work practices. Lab personnel can safeguard themselves from electrical risks by adhering to certain fundamental guidelines:
   a. Avoid contacting circuits with wet hands or wet materials
   b. All current-transmitting parts of any electrical devices must be enclosed
   c. Proper grounding of all electrical pieces of equipment
   d. All power outlets that could be exposed to wet conditions should be equipped with ground-fault circuit interrupters
   e. Switch off instruments, when not in use
   f. Safe work practices must be ensured

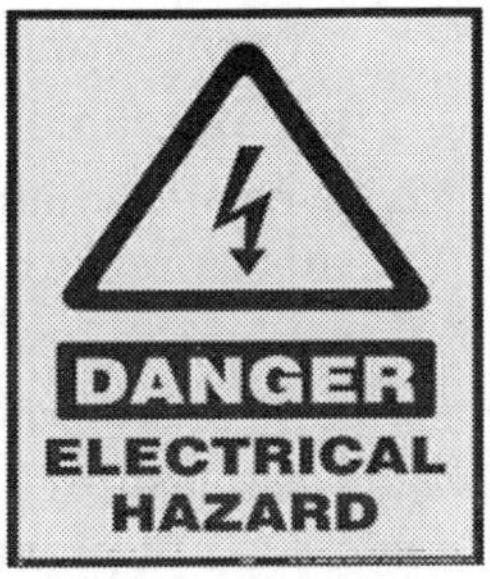

2. **Fire:** The danger of fire is always imminent as long as there are volatile, flammable solvents in the laboratory. The following precautions should be taken to prevent fire outbreaks:
   a. Use fire extinguishers at strategic locations in the laboratory
   b. Smoking should be prohibited in the laboratory
   c. Emergency exit should be present
   d. Avoid open flames in the laboratory
   e. All connections of flammable gases to instruments such as the flame photometer should be leak-proof
   f. Always work in a fume chamber when working with flammable solvents

3. **Equipment:** Laboratory personnel must be trained on the proper use of laboratory equipment before use. These general guidelines should be followed:
   a. Good operational and safety training must be practised
   b. Instructions provided in the manufacturer's manuals and standard operating procedures must be followed
   c. The centrifuge lid should be closed while operating it
   d. Do not operate the centrifuge without the rotor being properly balanced (as shown in the figure)
   e. Disinfect or clean all the laboratory machinery weekly
   f. Autoclave can cause burns and should be handled carefully with heating gloves

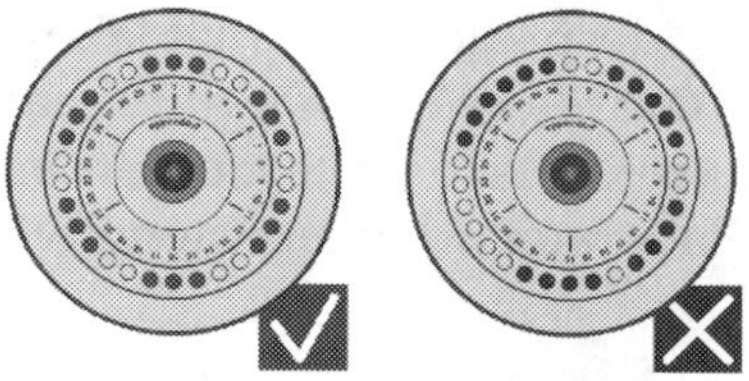
Balancing a centrifuge rotor

4. **Glassware:** Broken glassware should not be handled, any broken glassware, e.g. flasks, beakers and pipettes with broken tips should be discarded as they are a source of danger.

Chemical hazards: Chemical safety precautions are essential to prevent serious workplace injuries.

1. **Flammable chemicals:** In general, the flammability of a chemical is determined by its flash point, the lowest temperature at which an ignition source can cause the chemical to ignite momentarily under certain controlled conditions.
   a. Never heat flammable substances with an open flame
   b. Flammable chemicals like methanol, ethanol, and acetone must be stored in inflammable storage rooms or in inflammable storage cabinets
   c. Handle reactive chemicals with all proper safety precautions: Segregation in storage, prohibition of mixing even small quantities with other chemicals without prior approval
   d. Flammable chemicals must be stored in a cool place
2. **Corrosive chemicals:** Handle corrosive and contact-hazard chemicals with all proper safety precautions.
   a. Wear safety goggles and face shields, gloves, and a laboratory apron or lab coat
   b. Strong acids (sulphuric acid, nitric acid), and strong alkalis (sodium hydroxide, potassium hydroxide), must be handled very carefully
   c. Do not pipette liquids by mouth; use mechanical pipetting devices

3. **Toxic chemicals:** Emergency response planning and training are very important when working with highly toxic compounds.
   a. Avoid inhalation of toxic chemicals
   b. Wear protective gloves, booties, and a Tyvek® suit when necessary, while performing cleanup activities for toxic chemicals like cyanide, mercuric nitrate, formaldehyde.
   c. Face and eye protection is necessary to prevent ingestion, inhalation, and skin absorption of toxic chemicals.
   d. The cleanup of highly toxic substances should not be attempted alone
4. **Explosive chemicals:** Do not use explosive chemicals if less hazardous alternatives are possible.
   a. Store explosive wastes separately from other wastes.
   b. Fire-hazard chemicals must be used only in chemical hoods, away from sources of ignition, e.g. picric acid.
5. **Carcinogens:** Carcinogens are chronic toxins causing cancer, with long latency periods that can cause damage after repeated or long-duration exposures and often do not have immediate apparent harmful effects. When working with carcinogenic materials (benzidine, o-toluidine, ethidium bromide, etc.) in the laboratory be sure to:
   a. Wear a mask and gloves while handling.
   b. All procedures should take place in a controlled area, that is, clearly labelled with a warning and restricted access.
   c. Limit access to carcinogens, keep containers and amounts used as small as possible.
   d. Store in a designated area with the appropriate hazard signs and ventilation if required.

Biological hazards: For controlling biological hazards, the following points must be kept in mind:

a. Making sure biological hazards are kept in primary tubes and secondary storage boxes that will prevent leaks in the event of containment failure.
b. All samples from patients that are potentially infectious, e.g. HIV, HbsAg, Tb, must be handled carefully.
c. Dispose of biological hazardous chemicals as soon as possible.
d. Biological hazardous waste should not be allowed to accumulate.
e. Wherever possible dilute biological hazardous wastes in a safe solvent, since many wastes are more stable when diluted.

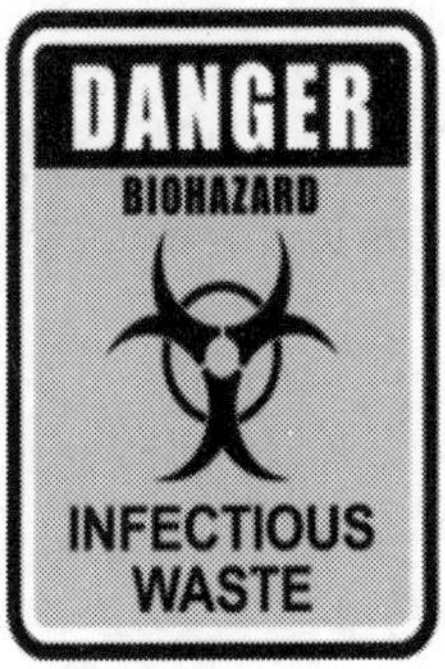

1. **Blood:** When handling blood samples, personnel need to:
   a. Wear two pairs of disposable gloves, the outsides of which should be thrown away and replaced
   b. Wear a lab coat, a mask, and an eye safety during every procedure
2. **Culture media:** When handling culture media:
   a. Proper hand washing to be done before and after the experiment.

b. Use an appropriate disinfectant to clean the work surfaces. Before using, inspect all the medium and reagents.
c. The cultures should be taken from authorized sources.
d. Acquire new microbe stock cultures every year
e. Always wear proper personal protection.

3. **Urine:**
a. Use protective laboratory coats and gloves.
b. Working with human material like urine, should be confined to a quiet, marked area with no or little interference from others.

4. **Stool:**
a. Wear adequate personal protective equipment (PPE).
b. When necessary, use biological safety cabinets.
c. Stool should be collected in a dry sterilized container and should be free from other body secretions like urine.
d. Daily decontaminate the working table and after any spill.

5. **Body fluids:**
a. PPE including gloves, lab coats, masks, and protective eyewear should be worn during body fluids examination.
b. Always maintain hand hygiene.
c. Regular sterilisation of all pieces of equipment.

Effluent Treatment Plan (ETP)

The liquid waste that is effluent from the instruments is a biomedical waste that has to be disinfected before releasing into the sewage.

Biomedical waste	*Disinfectant*
500 litres of biomedical waste	5 litres (1.25 litres of 1% sodium hypochlorite + 3.75 litres of distilled water)

Biomedical waste is treated with disinfectant in biomedical waste tank for a contact period of one hour and then released to sewage treatment plant (STP).

CHAPTER

2

Laboratory Safety Measures

First aid equipment in a lab: In the event of an emergency or accident in the lab, each laboratory should have the following first aid supplies, which should be clearly marked throughout the space. It is recommended to inspect and replace the first aid kit's components twice a year. The basic laboratory first aid kit should contain:

- 2% sodium bicarbonate
- 5% acetic acid
- Soap solution
- Antiseptic lotion
- Cotton
- Gauze
- Tape
- Scissors

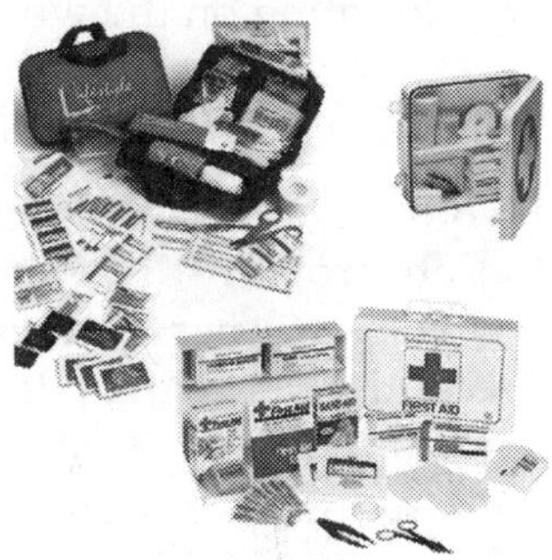

FIRST AID IN LABORATORY ACCIDENTS

1. Acid Burns

a. For at least 10 to 15 minutes, hold the affected area of skin under running water
b. Leave the wound exposed, and wait to apply any cream or ointment until professional medical assistance is available.
c. In case of accidents with strong acid first wash with water and then with dilute ammonia (1–2%) or sodium bicarbonate solution

2. Alkali Burns

a. Immediately rinse with a large amount of cool water. Rinsing within 1 minute of the burn can reduce the risk of complications. However, some alkali burns are made worse if rinsed (flushed) with water.
b. Wipe the skin with cotton soaked in 5% acetic acid
c. Visit the doctor for further assistance

3. Injury by Broken Glass

a. Wash immediately
b. Press on the bleeding
c. Apply an antiseptic lotion

4. Electric Shock

a. Put off the main switch.
b. Open the airways and check for breathing, if breathing is not normal, start chest compressions.
c. Call the doctor immediately.

Precautionary Measures

1. One has to be very careful while handling laboratory materials
2. Never pour water into acids
3. Keep acids on the lower shelf
4. Do not use broken glass
5. Label the poisonous chemicals
6. Fire extinguisher must be checked periodically
7. Keep a sand bucket
8. No smoking
9. No mouth pipetting
10. No eating on the workbench.

UNIVERSAL PRECAUTIONS TO AVOID INFECTIONS

Frequent hand washing, refraining from mouth pipetting, keeping food and drink out of the lab, properly disposing of biohazardous and medical waste, and using engineering controls and **personal protective equipment (PPE)** are all examples of universal precautions. The main techniques for limiting exposure include engineering controls, such as ventilation systems, and the use of biosafety cabinets. Examples of PPE include:

1. Use rubber gloves, nose mask
2. Use eye shield, face shield, apron
3. Hand washing
4. Sterilization/disinfection
5. Proper biomedical waste disposal

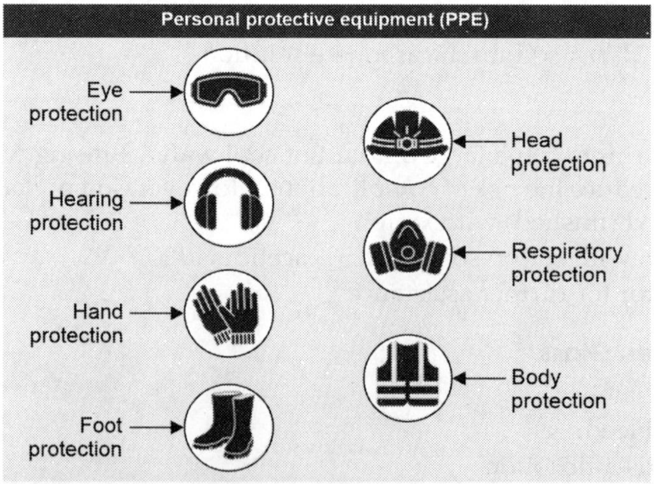

CHAPTER

3

Biomedical Waste Management

BIOMEDICAL WASTE

Biomedical waste encompasses any waste that arises during the diagnosis, treatment, or immunization processes of humans or animals, as well as from research activities. In healthcare facilities, proper management of biomedical waste is essential to ensure the safety of both personnel and the environment. The following guidelines for management of healthcare waste as per Biomedical Waste Management Rules, 2016 given by the Government of India outline the categorization, containment, and disposal methods for various types of biomedical waste:

Category	*Type of waste*	*Type of container*	*Treatment and disposal options*
Yellow	1. Human anatomical waste 2. Animal anatomical waste 3. Soiled waste like cotton, plaster, dressings contaminated with blood 4. Expired medicines 5. Chemical waste 6. Chemical liquid waste–separate collection system	Yellow colour plastic bag	Incineration Autoclaving + shredding
Red	Contaminated recyclable waste – IV set – Catheter – Urine bag – Gloves – Syringes	Red colour plastic bag	Autoclaving + shredding
White	Waste sharps and metals – Needles – Scalpels – Blades	Puncture proof containers	Autoclaving + shredding
Blue Autoclaving	a. Glassware – Broken glass vials, slides, ampoules b. Metallic body implants	Cardboard box with blue colour marking	Disinfection ↓ Sent for recycling

By adhering to these guidelines, healthcare facilities can effectively manage biomedical waste, minimise risks to public health and the environment, and ensure compliance with regulatory standards.

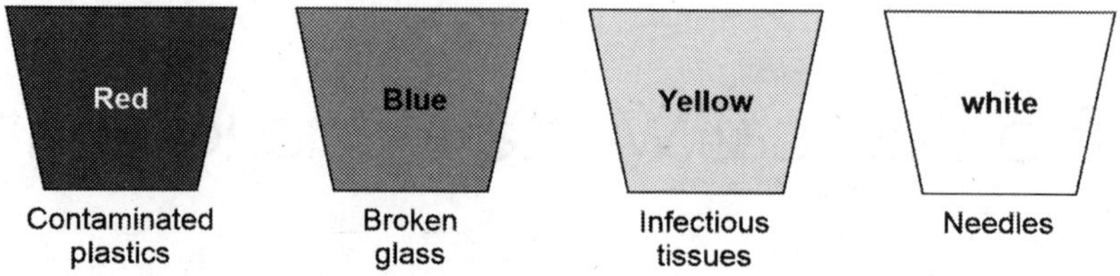

Colour coded bags for biomedical waste containers

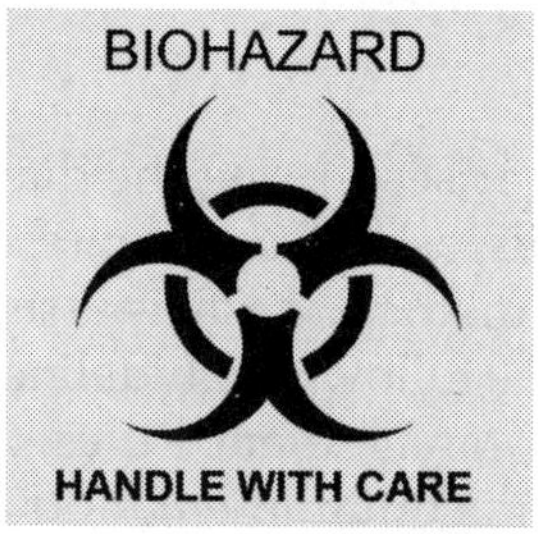

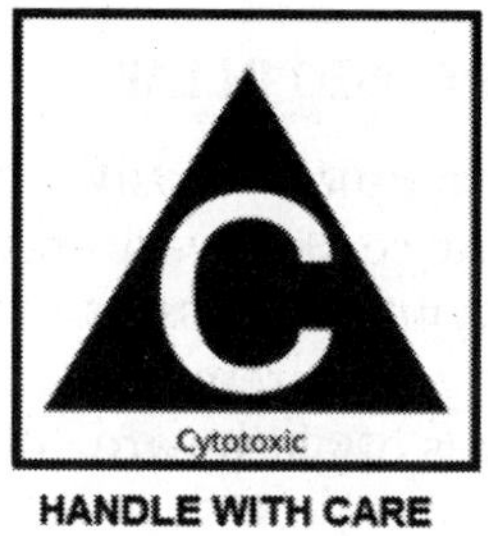

CHAPTER

4

Glasswares

TYPES OF GLASSWARE USED IN LABORATORIES

Glasswares are made up of borosilicate glass. Glassware is an integral component of laboratory equipment, serving various purposes in scientific experiments, analyses, and research. Different types of glassware are designed to meet specific laboratory needs, facilitating accurate measurements, reactions, and sample handling. Here are some commonly used types of glassware in laboratories:

Beakers

Beakers are cylindrical vessels with a flat bottom and a spout for pouring. They are used for mixing, heating, and holding liquids during experiments. Beakers come in various sizes, allowing for different volumes of liquids to be accommodated.

- Capacity from 5 to 5000 ml
- Used for the preparation of solutions

Flasks

Flasks, such as Erlenmeyer flasks and volumetric flasks, are used for measuring, mixing, and storing liquids. Erlenmeyer flasks have a conical shape with a narrow neck, ideal for swirling liquids without spilling, while volumetric flasks are calibrated to contain precise volumes of liquids.

Test Tubes

Test tubes are small, cylindrical containers used for holding, mixing, and heating small quantities of liquids or solids. They are often used in qualitative analysis, reaction observations, and small-scale experiment.

Pipettes

Pipettes are slender glass tubes with tapered tip used for transferring precise volumes of liquids. They come in various types, including volumetric pipettes for accurate measurements and micropipettes for handling small volumes with high precision.

Burettes

Burettes are long, graduated glass tubes with a stopcock at the bottom used for precise titration measurements. They allow for the controlled addition of a titrant to a solution until the reaction reaches its endpoint.

Graduated Cylinders

Graduated cylinders are tall, narrow containers with calibrated volume markings used for measuring and transferring liquids. They provide accurate volume measurements for solutions and are commonly used in quantitative analysis.

- Capacity 10–2000 ml
- Used to measure liquid

Desiccators

Desiccators are airtight containers used for storing moisture-sensitive substances under dry conditions. They typically consist of a glass jar with a removable lid and a desiccant, such as silica gel, to absorb moisture from the air inside the container.

Watch Glasses

Watch glasses are shallow, circular glass dishes used as covers for beakers or evaporating dishes. They can also be used for evaporation, crystallization, or as a surface for observing reactions.

Petri Dishes

Petri dishes are shallow, circular glass or plastic dishes with a lid used for culturing microorganisms, agar plates, and performing microbiological experiments. They provide a sterile environment for the growth and observation of microorganisms.

Funnel

Funnels are cone-shaped glassware used for transferring liquids from one container to another without spillage. They come in various sizes and shapes and are equipped with a narrow stem for precise pouring.

Each type of glassware serves a specific function in laboratory operations, contributing to the accuracy, efficiency, and safety of scientific experiments and analyses. Proper handling, cleaning, and maintenance of glassware are essential to ensure reliable results and prevent contamination in laboratory procedures.

General Glassware

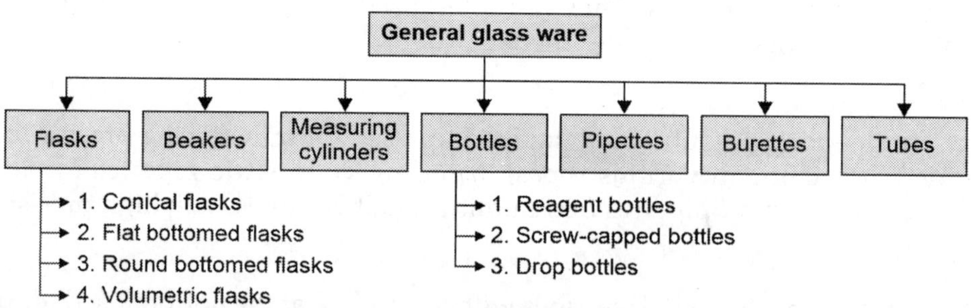

1. Beakers—capacity 25 to 5000 ml, used to make reagents.

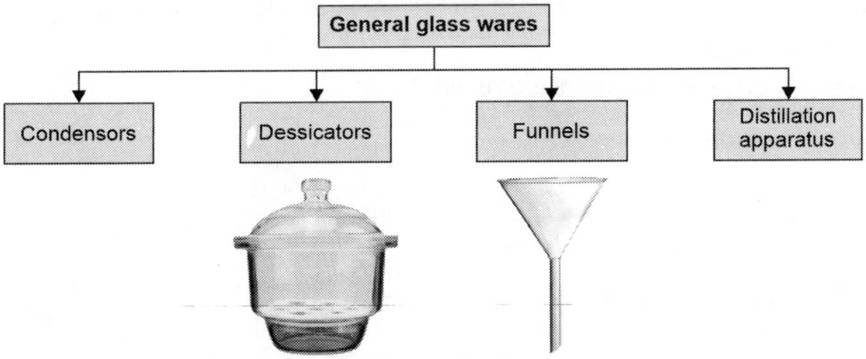

2. Flasks—capacity 25 to 5000 ml, used for heating

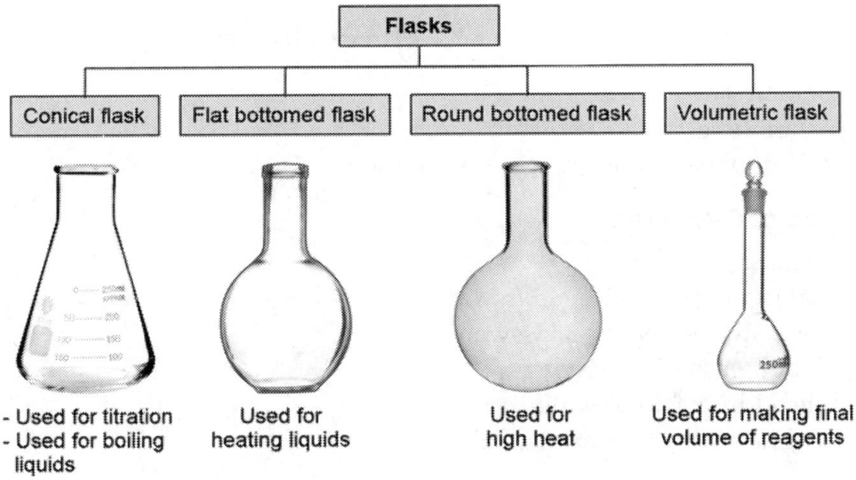

3. Measuring cylinders—capacity 10–2000 ml, used to measure liquids
4. Bottles
   – Screw-capped bottles—used to store hygroscopic reagents
   – Drop bottles—used for a drop of solutions

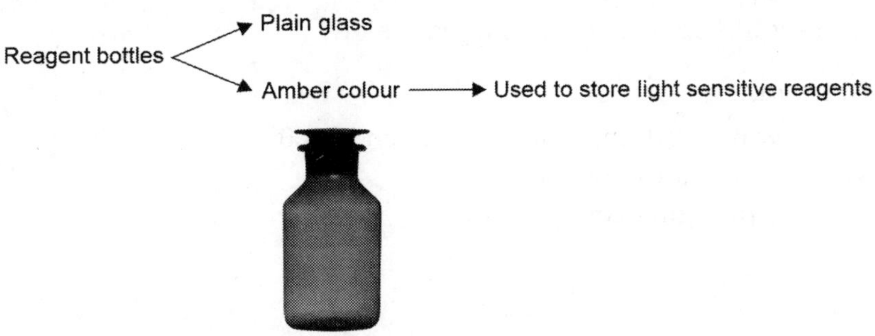

5. Pipettes
   Used for dispensing controlled quantity of liquids

6. Burettes
   – Used for titration
   – Used for dispensing corrosive reagents
7. Tubes

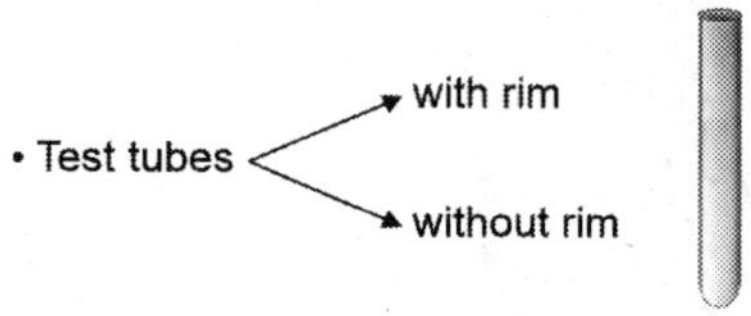

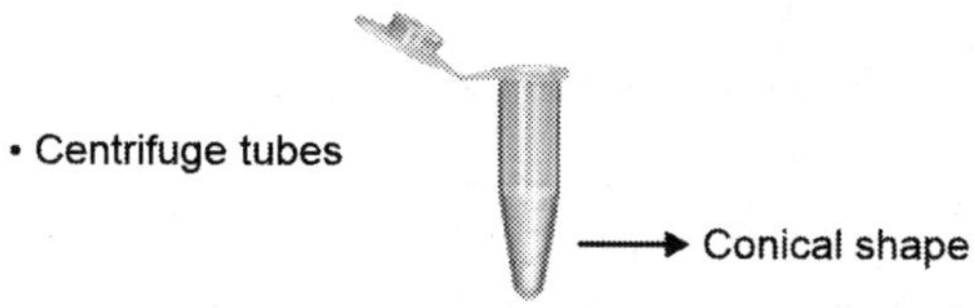

   – Digestion tubes
   – Folin Wu tubes → For glucose estimation

Maintenance of Glassware

1. Heat the glassware slowly
2. Use metal gauze for heating glassware
3. Use water bath for heating glassware
4. Cool the hot glassware slowly
5. Stir while adding acid to water
6. Use ice while adding water to alkali.

Cleaning of Glassware

1. Soak glassware in 1% HCl for long hours
2. Soak glassware in tap water immediately after use
3. Use nitric oxide to remove contaminated material
4. Scrub with detergents
5. Rinse thoroughly in tap water
6. Final rinse should always be in distilled water.

Drying of Glassware

1. Drain excess water and dry in a hot air oven at 100°C
2. Dry at room temperature on a towel
3. Avoid dust by plugging cotton.

CHAPTER

5

Blood Collection Techniques (Phlebotomy)

The technique of collecting blood samples from a peripheral vein is phlebotomy.

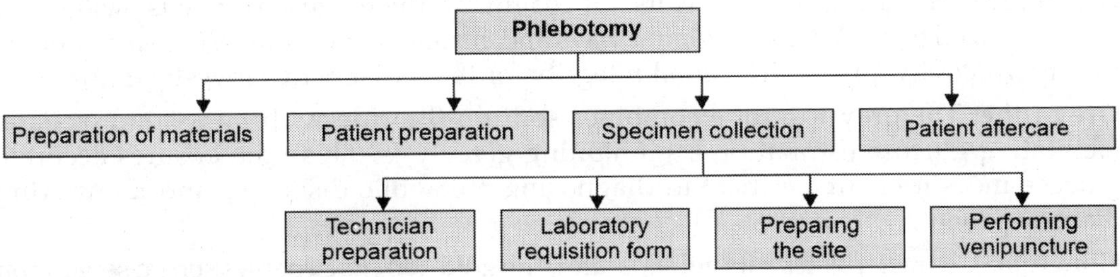

A. PREPARATION OF MATERIALS

- Disposable syringes and needles or vacutainers (19, 20, 22 G)
- Gauze pad/cotton
- Tourniquet
- 70% ethanol
- Needle and syringe disposing bins (white and red)

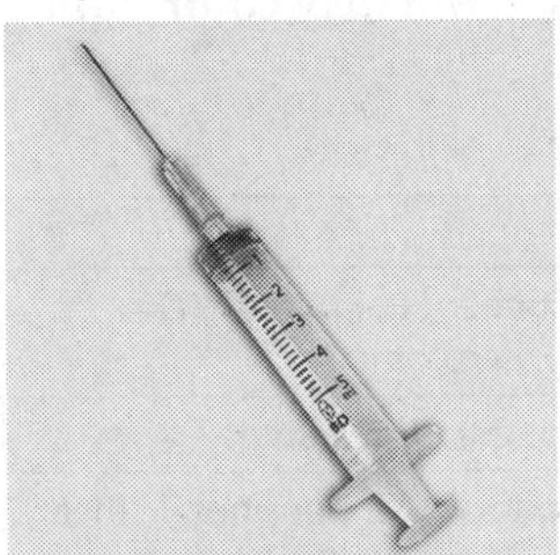
Syringe and needle

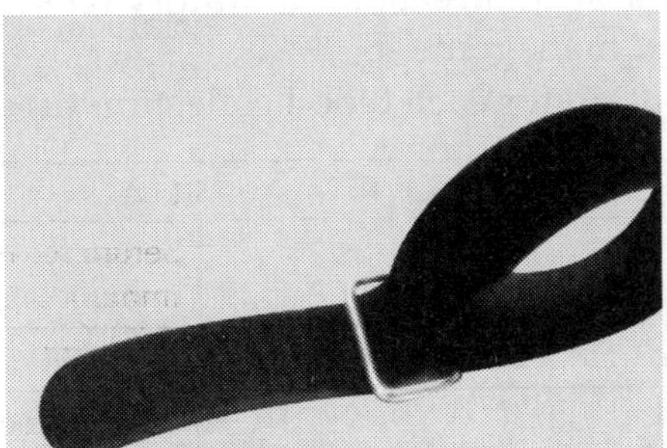
Tourniquet

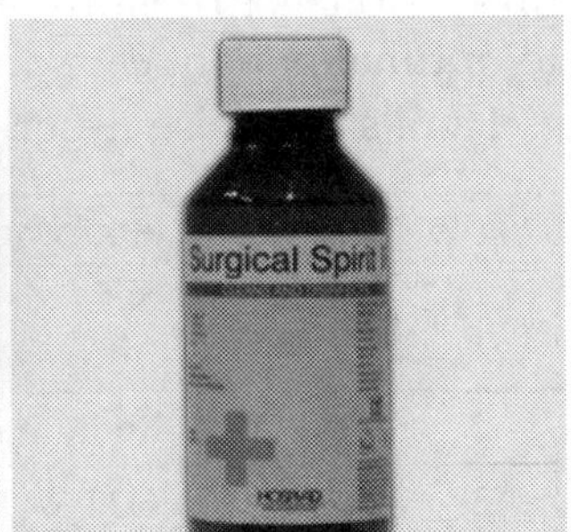

Spirit

Blood Collection Tubes

Blood collection tubes are indispensable tools in the realm of medical diagnostics, playing a crucial role in obtaining and preserving blood samples for various laboratory analyses. Each tube is uniquely designed, featuring specific additives tailored to stabilize blood components for different types of tests.

Red tube: The red-top tube, devoid of anticoagulants, is employed for serum collection. It serves as the vessel for biochemical parameter assessments, immunological assays, and serological investigations. Blood allowed to clot in these tubes yields clear serum, essential for diverse diagnostic procedures.

Blue tube: Recognizable by its blue stopper, this tube contains 3.2% sodium citrate, an anticoagulant crucial for coagulation studies. It is instrumental in measuring clotting factors, facilitating tests such as prothrombin time (PT) and activated partial thromboplastin time (APTT), pivotal in assessing hemostasis.

Lavender tube: The lavender-top tube, incorporating EDTA (ethylene diamine tetra acetic acid), is tailored for the collection of whole blood. EDTA prevents blood clotting by chelating calcium ions, rendering it ideal for complete blood count (CBC) analyses and peripheral blood smear evaluations, vital for hematological assessments.

Green tube: Featuring heparin as its anticoagulant, the green-top tube is designated for specialized tests such as troponin assays and chromosome studies. Heparin inhibits thrombin activity, preserving blood integrity for these distinctive investigations.

Grey tube: The grey-top tube combines sodium fluoride with potassium oxalate, facilitating glucose estimation by inhibiting glycolysis. This tube ensures accurate glucose measurements, critical in diagnosing metabolic disorders and monitoring diabetic patients.

Gold tube: Characterized by its gel separator, the gold-top tube enables serum separation from clotting blood. This facilitates biochemical analyses and microbiological assays, providing clear serum samples free from cellular contaminants for precise testing.

Black tube: Utilizing 3.8% sodium citrate, the black-top tube serves as the vessel for erythrocyte sedimentation rate (ESR) determinations. It stabilizes blood samples, allowing erythrocytes to settle, aiding in the assessment of inflammatory conditions.

In summary, blood collection tubes are indispensable tools in modern medicine, facilitating accurate diagnostic testing across a spectrum of medical disciplines. Understanding their distinct compositions and applications is essential for healthcare professionals to ensure precise and reliable laboratory results, ultimately contributing to optimal patient care and management.

Here's a concise description for each blood collection tube.

S. No	*Colour*	*Anticoagulant*	*Use*
1	Red	Nil	Serum for biochemical parameters, immunology, serology
2	Blue	Sodium citrate 3.2%	PT, APTT, coagulation studies
3	Lavender	EDTA	Whole blood for CBC, peripheral smear, HbA1c
4	Green	Heparin	Troponin, chromosome studies
5	Grey	Sodium fluoride + potassium oxalate	Glucose estimation
6	Gold	Serum separator tube with gel	Biochemistry, microbiology
7	Black	Sodium citrate 3.8%	ESR

B. PATIENT PREPARATION

1. Patient must not drink tea/coffee for fasting sample
2. Patient must relax for at least 15 minutes before blood collection
3. Ask for any bleeding tendency in patients

Position the patient

↓

Sit comfortably in a chair

↓

The arm should be straight and extended on a slanting armrest

↓

Do not bend the elbow

↓

The patient can lie down on a couch comfortably if the patient wants

C. SPECIMEN COLLECTION

1. Technician Preparation

Pleasant approach to patients

↓

Confirm the identity of the patient

↓

PPE: Wear gloves, apron, face mask, face shield, etc.

↓

Do the procedure properly, and quickly without discomfort to patients

↓

Keep the tubes labelled

2. Laboratory Requisition Form

1. Complete request form must have:
   - Patient full name, age, sex
   - OP/IP number
   - List of required tests
   - Date and time of collection
   - Ward/department
   - Name of the physician/signature
   - Diagnosis of the clinical condition
   - Medication/treatment details

3. Preparing the Site

Select the vein-median cubital vein (common)

↓

Cephalic or basilic vein if needed

↓

Do not try ankle or foot veins

↓

Avoid healed burn areas

↓

Feel the vein with the tip of your fingers—bounce, direction, depth of the vein

↓

Apply the tourniquet briefly

↓

Clean the area with spirit cotton in a circular fashion from centre to outside

↓

Allow it to dry in the air

↓

Do not touch the site after cleaning

↓

Check the syringe and needle

↓

Check the piston of the syringe

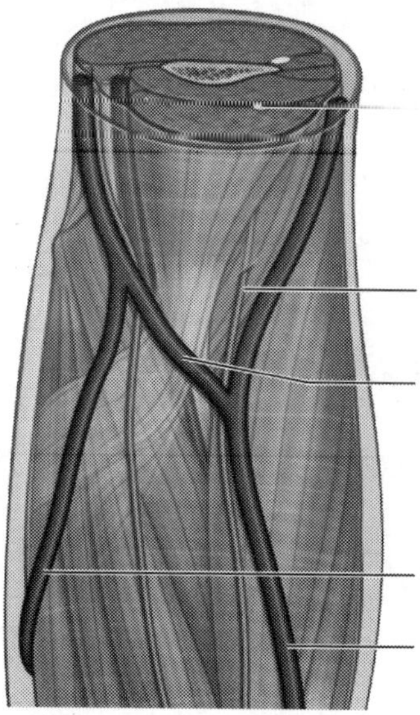

Veins of upper limb

4. Perform Venipuncture

Hold the patient's arm tight and stretch the skin with thumb

↓

Penetrate the vein at 30°–40° angle

↓

The resistance will be released when needle enters the vein

↓

Remove the tourniquet

↓

Do not penetrate deeper

↓

Draw adequate quantity of blood for all the tubes

↓

Press a cotton ball on punctured site and remove the needle

↓

Tell patients to keep elbow flexed till bleeding stops

↓

Put the blood sample in tubes after removing needle from syringe

↓

Mix the tubes by gentle inversion (5–6 times)

↓

Dispose syringe and needle in BMW bins correctly

D. PATIENT AFTERCARE

1. If bleeding continues for a long time apply a pressure bandage and elevate the arm.
2. If the patient feels dizzy—ask them to lie down flat.
3. Inform the physician if needed.

NOT TO DO

1. Do not make more than 2 attempts in pricking.
2. Do not collect blood above the IV line site.
3. Do not collect from any other site other than the upper arm.
4. Do not do arterial puncture.
5. Ask the help of seniors or doctors for blood collection in pediatric children.

CHAPTER

6

Anticoagulants and Vacutainers

1. Sodium Fluoride

- Weak anticoagulant
- Inhibits glycolysis
- Used for glucose estimation
- Should not be used for the estimation of urea, enzymes

2. Heparin

- Sodium, potassium salts
- Inhibits factor X
- Antithrombin III activity
- Should not be used for the estimation of electrolytes, thyroid function test

3. Ethylene Diamine Tetra Acetic Acid (EDTA)

- Used for hematology
- Inhibits coagulation by binding calcium
- Should not be used for the estimation of electrolytes, ALP, CK, calcium, iron

4. Citrate

- Used for coagulation studies
- Used for estimation of PT, APTT
- Should not be used for the estimation of AST, ALT, ALP, calcium, phosphorus
- Reversible coagulation

5. Oxalates

- Inhibits coagulation by forming a complex with calcium
- Used for glucose estimation
- Should not be used for the estimation of ALP, amylase, LDH

Blood Collection Tubes (Vacutainers)			
S. No	*Colour*	*Anticoagulant*	*Use*
1	Red	Nil	Biochemical parameters, immunology, serology
2	Blue	Sodium citrate 3.2%	PT, APTT, coagulation studies
3	Lavender	EDTA	CBC, peripheral smear, HbA1c
4	Green	Heparin	Troponin, chromosome studies
5	Grey	Sodium fluoride + potassium oxalate	Glucose estimation
6	Gold	Serum separator tube with gel	Biochemistry, microbiology
7	Black	Sodium citrate 3.8%	ESR

CHAPTER

7

24 Hours Urine Collection and Urine Preservatives

24 Hours Urine Collection Procedure

Give a five-litre can to the patient with the label

↓

Add urine preservative to the can (5 ml of toluene)

↓

Fix a date for urine collection

↓

The morning 6 a.m. sample on that date must be discarded

↓

Following, all urine passed in that day for 24 hours must be collected

↓

Collect urine in a clean jar and pour it into the can

↓

Close the lid and keep it in the refrigerator (if no preservatives)

↓

The next day morning, at 6 am urine must be collected in the can

↓

Bring the sample to the lab

↓

Lab technician must measure the total volume of urine in the can

↓

Stir well and take a small sample of urine from the can for analysis

Tests Done in 24 Hours Urine

1. 24 hours urine protein = Urine volume × urine microprotein

Example: Urine volume = 1500 ml = 15 dL
Urine microprotein = 20 mg/dL
24 hours urine protein = 15 × 20 = 300 mg/day

2. 24 hours urine calcium, electrolytes, oxalates, uric acid, phosphates, pH.

Urine Preservatives

1. Boric acid
2. Hydrochloric acid
3. Acetic acid
4. Toluene
5. Thymol
6. Formalin

Urine Preservatives

1. Decrease bacterial contamination
2. Preserve the chemical constituents
3. Preserve the cells and casts in urine

CHAPTER

8

Types of Solutions

1. Saturated solution
2. Percent solution
3. Molar solution
4. Molal solution
5. Normal solution
6. Standard solution

Saturated Solution

- Solvent-liquid
- Solute-salt/chemical

The solute is continuously dissolved in solvent until a small amount of crystal is visible.

Example: Ammonium sulphate dissolved in water till saturation.

Percent Solution

It is prepared by dissolving 1 gram of substance in 100 ml of solvent
w/v → weight by volume
v/v → volume by volume

Example: 0.9% NaCl → 0.9 g of NaCl in 100 ml water, i.e. 900 mg of NaCl in 100 ml water.

Molar Solution

A molar solution is where a gram molecular weight of the substance is dissolved in a litre of solution.

$$1\text{ M} = \frac{\text{1 gram molecular weight of substance}}{\text{1 litre of solution}}$$

Example: Molecular weight of NaOH → Na = 23
O = 16
H = 1
Total = 40

$$1\text{ M NaOH} = \frac{\text{40 gram of NaOH}}{\text{1 litre of } H_2O}$$

Molal Solution

A molal solution is where 1 gram of molecular weight of the substance is dissolved in 1 kg of solvent.

$$1 \text{ molal} = \frac{1 \text{ gram molecular weight of the substance}}{1 \text{ kg of solvent}}$$

Example:

$$1 \text{ molal NaOH} = \frac{40 \text{ gram of NaOH}}{1 \text{ kg of } H_2O}$$

Understanding molal solutions is essential in various fields including chemistry, biochemistry, and pharmacology, where precise measurements of concentrations are required for accurate experimentation and analysis.

Normal Solution (N)

A gram equivalent weight of a substance dissolved in one litre of its solution is called a normal solution.

$$1 \text{ N} = \frac{\text{Equivalent weight of substance}}{1 \text{ litre of water}}$$

Normality is particularly useful in acid–base titrations and redox reactions, where the reaction stoichiometry involves the transfer of a fixed number of equivalents of one species to another. By expressing concentrations in terms of normality, it becomes easier to predict and calculate the quantities of reactants required for a specific reaction.

It is important to note that normality can only be directly compared between solutions that undergo the same type of reaction. For example, the normality of an acid solution cannot be directly compared to the normality of a solution involved in a redox reaction. However, within a given reaction type, normality provides a straightforward measure of concentration that simplifies stoichiometric calculations.

Standard Solution

The standard solution is the known concentration of a substance in a solution.

Uses

1. Used for preparing a standard graph
2. Used for estimating unknown concentration

Example: Standard solution of glucose, urea, creatinine, and albumin used in autoanalysers for calibration.

CHAPTER

9

Buffers and pH Indicators

BUFFERS

Buffers are solutions that do not change pH with the addition of a small amount of acid or alkali.

Buffer = Weak acid + salt of weak acid (or)
Weak base + salt of a weak base

Examples:
1. Phosphate buffer
2. Acetate buffer
3. Tris-HCl buffer

1. Phosphate buffer = Sodium dihydrogen phosphate (NaH_2PO_4)
+
Disodium hydrogen phosphate (Na_2HPO_4)
2. Acetate buffer = Acetic acid + sodium acetate
3. Tris HCl buffer = Tris + hydrochloric acid

Uses

Buffered substrates are used for the estimation of enzymes.

Indicators

Indicators are solutions that show one colour when ionised and a different colour when not ionised.

$$\underset{\text{(colour A)}}{\text{H indicator}} \rightleftharpoons H^+ + \underset{\text{(colour B)}}{\text{Indicator}}$$

Example: Phenolphthalein indicator
(1 gm phenolphthalein in 100 ml of 95% ethanol)

List of pH Indicators

S. No	*Indicator*	*Colour in acid*	*Colour in alkali*	*pH range*
1	Phenolphthalein	Colourless	Pink	8.3–10
2	Litmus	Red	Blue	4.5–8
3	Methyl red	Red	Yellow	4.4–6.2
4	Methyl orange	Red	Orange	3–4.4
5	Bromocresol green	Yellow	Green	3–4.6

Uses

1. Indicators are used to indicate changes in pH
2. Used as dyes in electrophoresis (bromophenol blue)
3. Used in the estimation of proteins (bromocresol green, pyrogallol red).

CHAPTER

10

Quality Control

QUALITY

- Ensures reliability
- Satisfy the needs of the customer.

Quality in Lab

1. Right test
2. Right person
3. Right method
4. Right report
5. Right time
6. Right cost

Error

Unavoidable but can be minimised

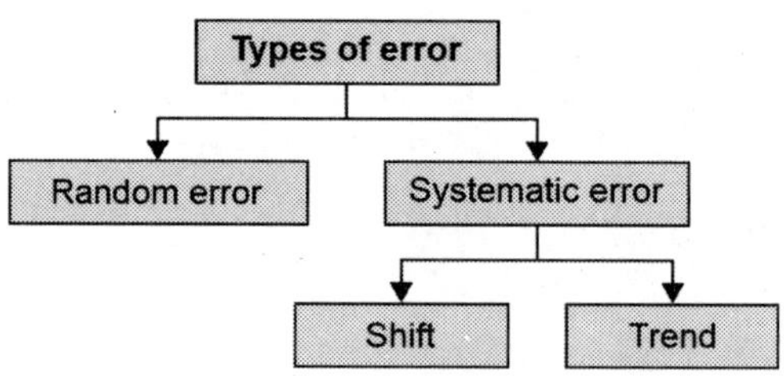

Accuracy

Closeness to the true value

Precision

Repeatability of the result

Sensitivity

The test can detect even a minimal quantity of the substance

Specificity

The test will detect only the specific substance

Control Material

- Lyophilised
- Stable for a long time
- Matrix similar to serum
- Level 1, level 2, level 3 controls

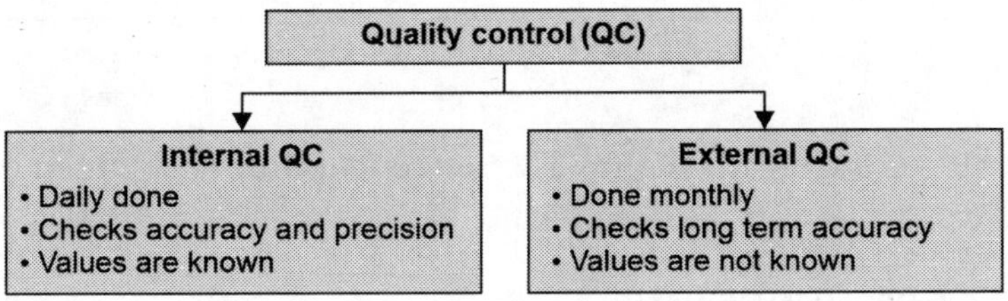

Control charts

- Levey - Jennings Chart
- Westgard's rule.

CHAPTER

11

Reference Ranges

The reference value is the normal value. The reference value is obtained from reference individuals.

ESTABLISHMENT OF REFERENCE VALUE

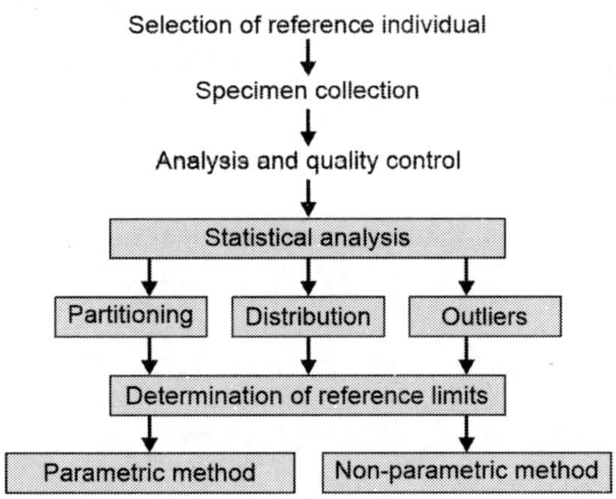

Use of Reference Value

- Reference value must be given in the report
- High values and low values must be flagged
- Reference value for age, sex, and weeks of pregnancy must be given.

CHAPTER

12

Calibration

- Calibration is setting the instrument right for testing
- Calibration is done for:
  1. New method
  2. New test
  3. QC out of range
- Calibration is done using:
  1. Standard solution
  2. Multical with known concentration
- Calibration is of two types:
  1. Single standard calibration (in semiauto-analysers)
  2. 5 points calibration (in automated analysers)

Calibration Procedure

1. Multical reconstitution
2. Setting the standard graph
3. Quality control check

I. Multical Reconstitution

Multical in lyophilised form

↓

Add 3 ml of distilled water to the vial

↓

Aliquot as 100 μl or 200 μl into eppendorf vials

↓

Store it in –20°C or –40°C in a deep freezer

↓

Take one vial for use each day

II. Setting the Standard Graph (e.g. ERBA XL 640)

Go to the QC/calibration option

↓

Select S_1 → test name

↓

Select S_2 → multical test name

↓

Select the QC test name

↓

Schedule OK

↓

START in the status monitor

III. QC (Quality Control) Check

- QC must be within ±2 SD
- Mean value must be achieved.

SECTION

II

Laboratory Instrumentation

1. pH Meter
2. Balances
3. Pipettes
4. Centrifuge
5. Colorimeter
6. Spectrophotometer
7. Autoanalysers
8. Electrophoresis
9. Chromatography
10. Estimation of Electrolytes
11. Arterial Blood Gas (ABG) Analyser
12. Enzyme-linked Immunosorbent Assay (ELISA)
13. Radioimmunoassay (RIA)

CHAPTER

1

pH Meter

Uses

pH meter—measures the pH of a solution.

$$pH = \frac{1}{\log [H^+]}$$

pH is a measure of the acidity or alkalinity of a solution.

$$0 \xrightarrow{\text{Acid}} 7 \xrightarrow{\text{Alkali}} 14$$

$$\uparrow$$

Neutral pH

PRINCIPLE

Potentiometry

The potential difference between two electrodes in a solution depends on the pH of the solution that is measured using a potentiometer.

Parts of a pH Meter

1. Glass electrode
2. Calomel reference electrode (KCl)
3. Platinum wires
4. Ag-AgCl
5. HCl (0.1N)

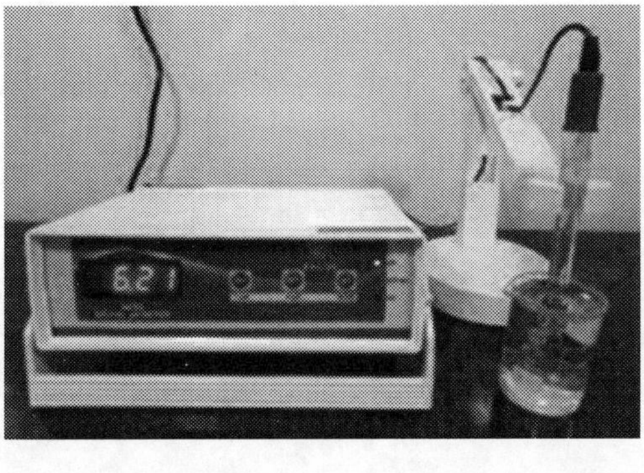

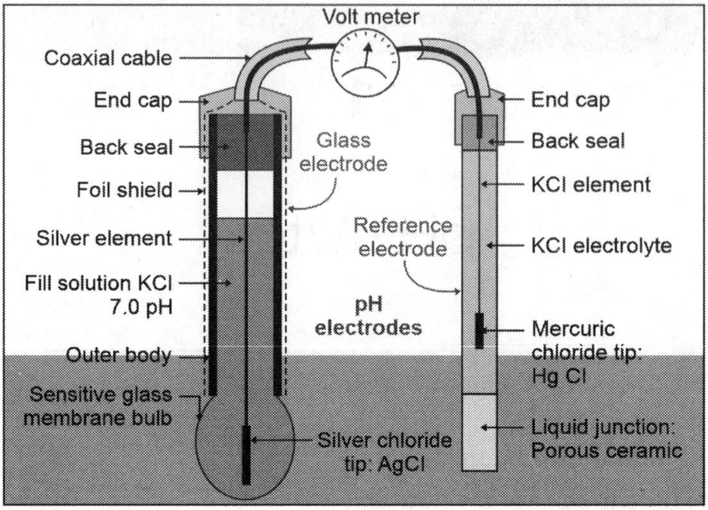

Combined electrode: The reference electrode and measuring electrode are combined in the pH meter.

Care and Maintenance

1. Electrode must be always dipped in water when not in use
2. Glass electrode must be clean
3. New electrodes must be dipped in 0.1 N HCl overnight for regeneration
4. The solution must be at room temperature.

CHAPTER

2

Balances

A balance is used to find out the mass of a substance.

TYPES

1. Physical balance
2. Analytical balance

Physical Balance

This is less accurate. Used for preparation of qualitative reagents

Analytical Balance

1. It is very accurate and highly sensitive
2. It is of two types: (a) Two-pan analytical balance, and (b) monopan balance
3. Used for preparation of analytical reagents

Components

1. Beam
2. Stirrups
3. Scale pans
4. Pointer
5. Ivory scale
6. Rigid supports
7. Handle
8. Central vertical pillar
9. Levelling screws

Weighing Procedure

1. Adjust the levelling screws to make the pillar vertical
2. Adjust the pointer to swing equally on both sides
3. Place the standard weight on one pan and the object to be weighed on the other pan and adjust

Monopan Balance

These are electronically operated and work on the principle of substitution of weights.

1. High accuracy and sensitivity
2. Quick weighing
3. Easy handling

4. Direct reading without the use of weights
5. Accuracy range 0.1 to 0.01 mg.

Electrical Balance

1. A null detector
2. A feedback loop
3. A read-out device.

Care and Maintenance

1. The balance should not be loaded with weight more than its maximum
2. The substance should not be weighed out
3. The cabinet of the balance should be kept closed while taking a reading
4. Clean the balance after use
5. Cover the balance when not in use
6. Do not spill the chemicals on the pan.

Performance and Quality Control

It is judged by:

1. Sensitivity
2. Precision
3. Accuracy

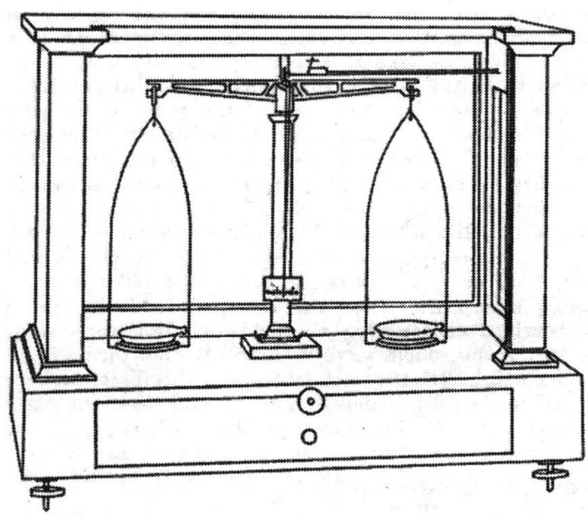

Two-pan analytical balance

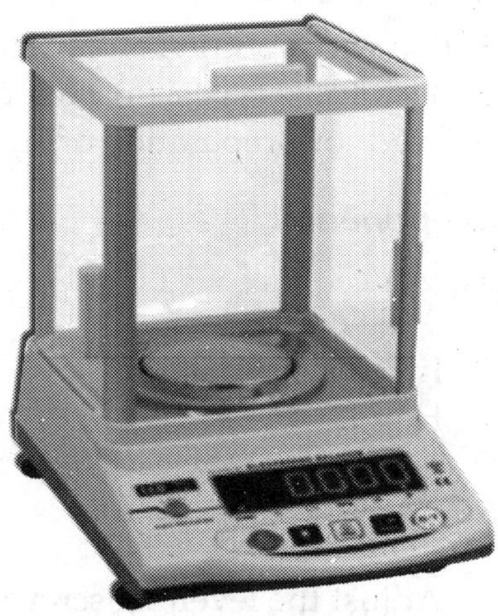

Electronic balance

CHAPTER 3

Pipettes

Pipettes are used to measure and deliver a volume of fluid.

TYPES

- TC—to contain
- TD—to deliver

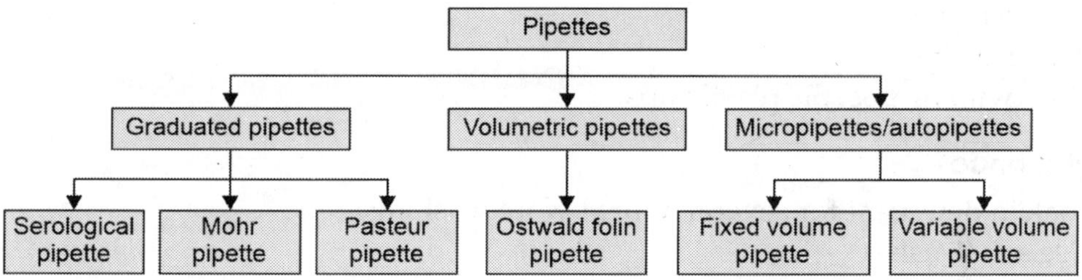

Serological Pipette

1. 0.1 ml to 10 ml
2. Graduated till tip
3. Blow out pipettes
4. Used for serological tests

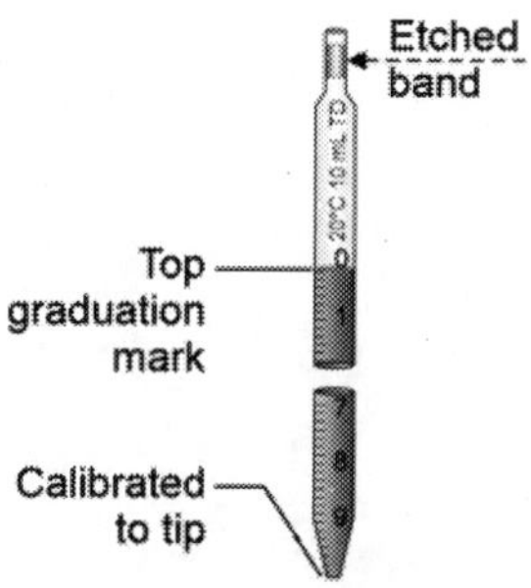

Serological pipette

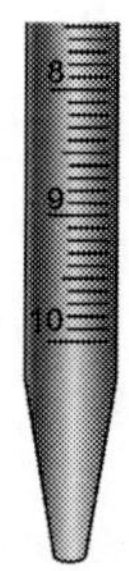

Mohr pipette

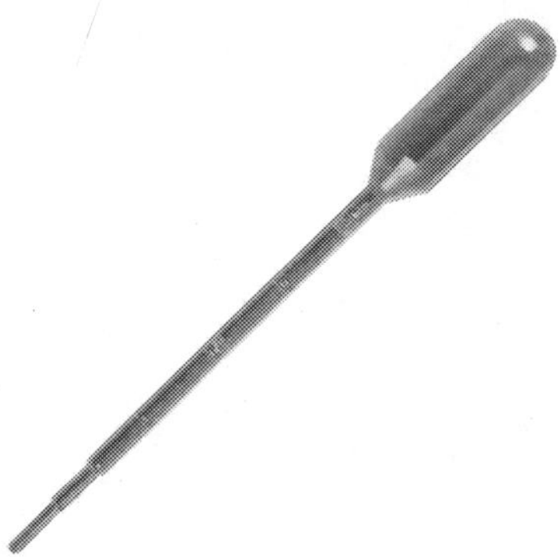

Pasteur pipette

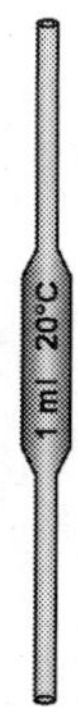

Ostwald folin pipette

Mohr Pipette

1. Not graduated till tip
2. Can be used for distilled water and reagents

Pasteur Pipette

1. Used to deliver drops of reagents
2. Rubber bulb attached to glass pipette

Volumetric Pipette

1. Have a bulb in the centre
2. Not graduated
3. Used only to deliver a specific volume
4. For example, Ostwald–Folin pipette

Micropipette

1. Available as fixed and variable volume pipettes
2. Fixed Volume—10 µL, 50 µL, 100 µL
3. Variable volume—10 to 100 µL, 100 to 1000 µL
4. Used for accurate measurements
5. Very sensitive
6. Autoclavable
7. Used with disposable plastic tips.

Maintenance

1. Soak in detergent for several hours before washing
2. Use soft brushes
3. Use mild acids to remove stains
4. Finally rinse in distilled water.

CHAPTER

4

Centrifuge

Centrifugation—separation technique used in the laboratory.

Principle

Centrifugal force–force acting from centre to periphery

$$S = V/\omega^2 r$$

S—Sedimentation coefficient
V—Migration
ω—Angular velocity
R—Radius

Components of a Centrifuge

1. Rotor
2. Cups/tubes
3. Motor
4. Timer

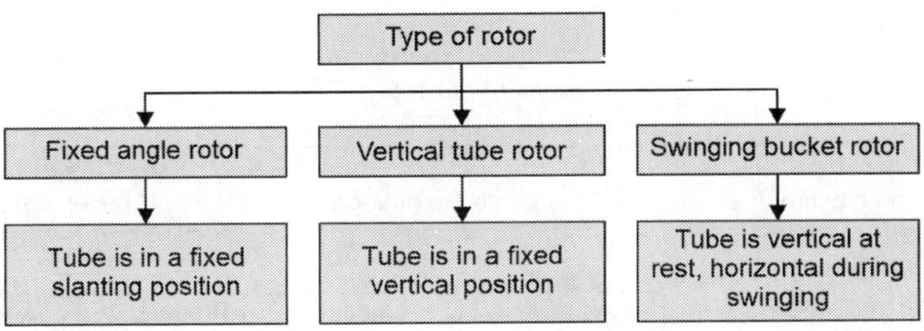

Small Bench Centrifuge

- Simple, less expensive
- Maximum 4000–6000 rpm

Large-capacity Refrigerated Centrifuge

- Have refrigerated rotor chambers
- Maximum speed of 6000 rpm

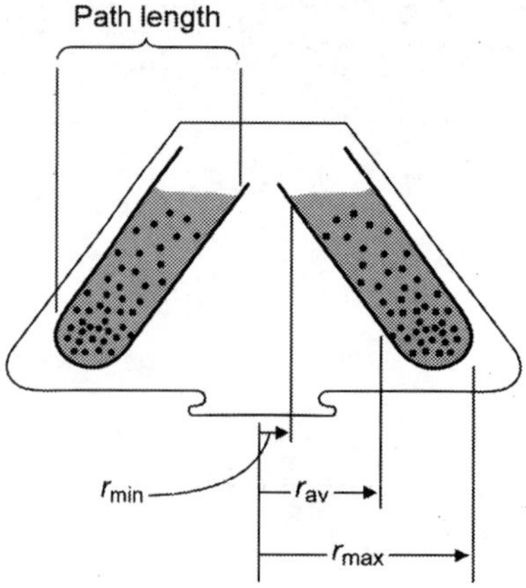

Fixed angle rotor

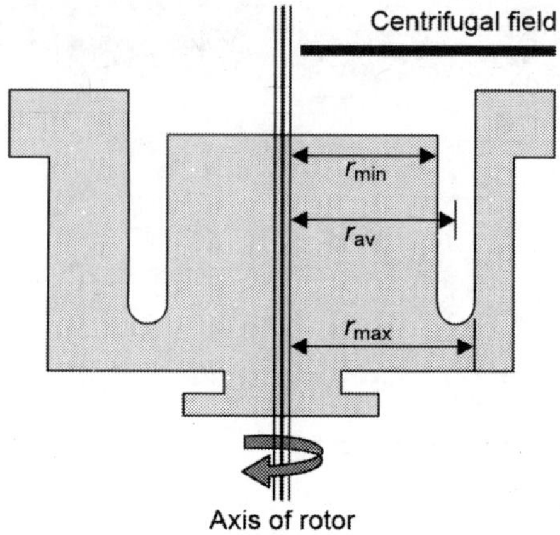

Vertical tube rotor

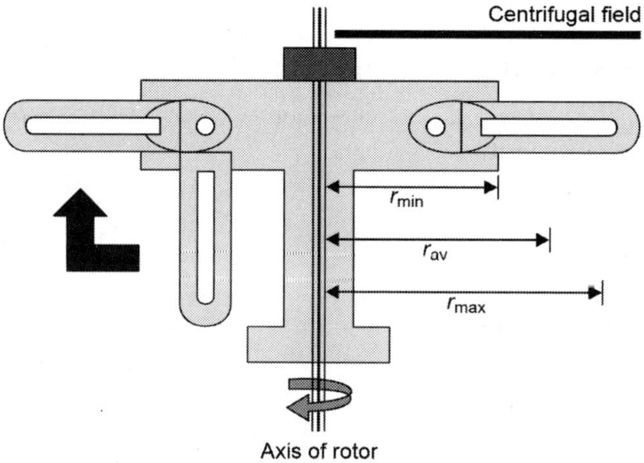

Swinging bucket rotor

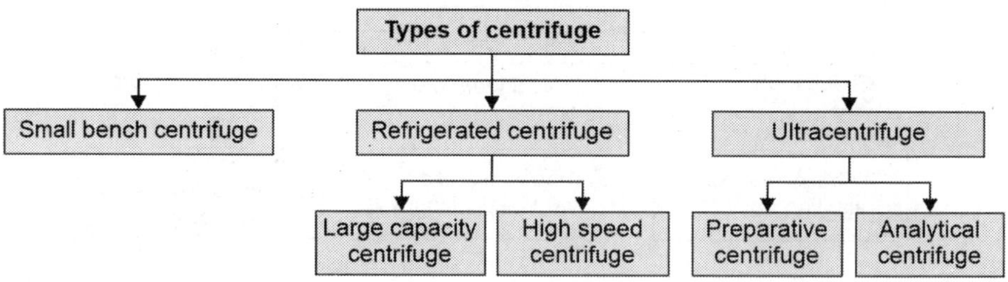

High-speed Refrigerated Centrifuge

Maximum rotor speed of 25,000 rpm

Preparative Ultracentrifuge

- Maximum speed of 80,000 rpm
- Sensitive temperature control

Analytical Ultracentrifuge

- Maximum speed of 70,000 rpm
- Used to analyze pure macromolecules

Uses

1. Separation of serum/plasma
2. Separation of protein free filtrate
3. Separation of subcellular organelles
4. Determination of molecular weight

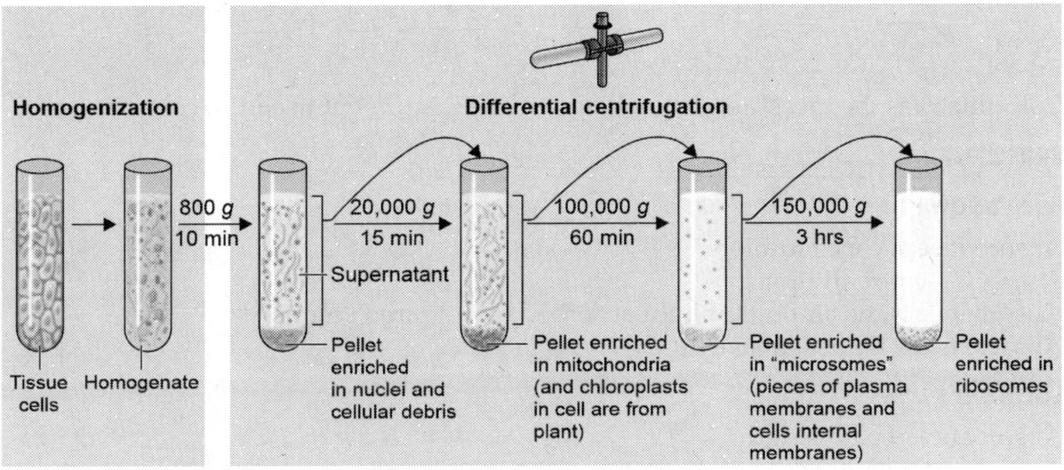

Separation of subcellular organelles

Care and Maintenance

1. Keep the centrifuge on a firm base
2. Do not keep the centrifuge near sensitive equipment
3. Balance the tubes/cups of the centrifuge
4. Close the lid tight
5. Clean the chamber and any spills
6. Replace graphite brush when needed
7. Check the temperature in a refrigerated centrifuge
8. Check the timer of the centrifuge using a stop clock.

CHAPTER

5

Colorimeter

Colorimetry is the measurement of colours. The instrument used is a colorimeter.

PRINCIPLE

Beer's Law

Absorbance $\propto$ concentration
$A \propto C$, C—concentration
Absorbance is the amount of light absorbed by coloured solution
Absorbance = Optical density (OD)

Lambert's Law

Absorbance $\propto$ path length
$A \propto l$, l–path length
$A \propto 1/T$, T—transmittance

Parts of a Colorimeter

1. Light source
2. Filter
3. Cuvette—sample holder
4. Photocell (detector)
5. Digital display

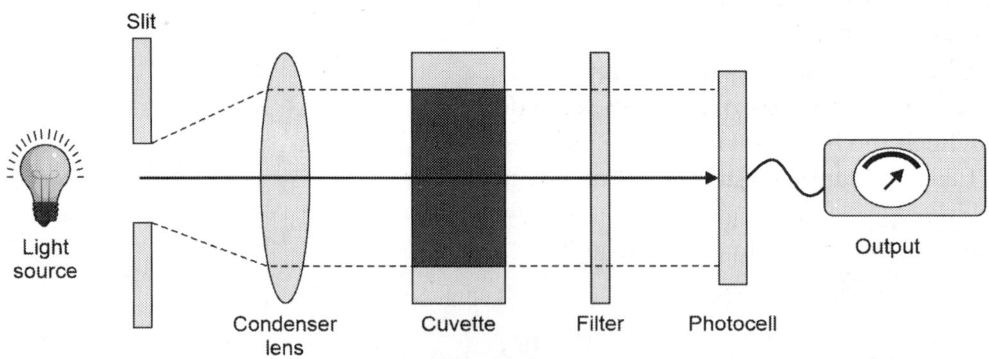

Parts of a colorimeter

Light Source

- Tungsten lamp
- Gives visible wavelength (400–700 nm)

Filter

- Colour filters
- Prism
- Grating

Colour of filter	*Wavelength (nm)*	*Colour of solution*
Violet	420	Brown
Blue	470	Yellowish brown
Green	520	Pink
Yellow	580	Purple
Red	680	Green

Cuvette

- Glass/quartz cuvette
- Fill 3/4th of the tube
- Cylindrical/square/rectangular

Photocell

- Convert light energy into electrical energy
- Photomultiplier tubes are also used

Digital display

The electrical signal is amplified, recorded and displayed as OD or T.

Uses

1. Quantitative estimation of analytes, e.g. glucose, urea, creatinine, cholesterol
2. Estimation of enzyme assays

Procedure

- Prepare three solutions B, S, T
  - B—blank
  - S—standard (known concentration)
  - T—test (unknown concentration)
- Switch on the instrument
- Choose the colour filter
- Adjust OD to zero
- Pour the sample into a cuvette and place it inside
- Take the readings as OD.

Calculation

$$\text{Concentration} = \frac{\text{OD of test} - \text{OD of blank}}{\text{OD of standard} - \text{OD of blank}} \times \text{Conc. of standard}$$

CHAPTER

6

Spectrophotometer

An instrument used to measure coloured solutions.

Principle

- Beer's law
- Lambert's law

PARTS OF A SPECTROPHOTOMETER

1. Light source
2. Entrance slit
3. Prism
4. Exit slit
5. Cuvette
6. Photodetector
7. Digital display

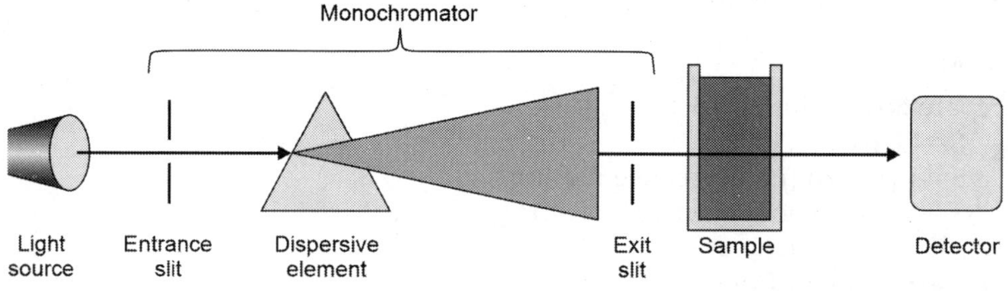

Parts of a spectrophotometer

Light source

- Hydrogen lamp
- Halogen lamp

Prism

- Diffraction grating or prism is used
- Wavelength is separated by adjusting slit
- Glass or quartz prism

Cuvettes

- Quartz thermocuvettes used for UV light
- Plastic cuvettes are also used
- Cylindrical or rectangular

Photodetectors

Photocells and phototubes are used

Display

Read out %T, OD or mg/dL

Uses

1. Quantitative estimation of analytes, e.g. glucose, urea, creatinine, cholesterol
2. Estimation of enzyme assays
3. Used to measure porphyrins

Procedure

1. Prepare three solutions B, S, T
   - B—blank
   - S—standard (known concentration)
   - T—test (unknown concentration)
2. Switch on the instrument
3. Choose the colour filter
4. Adjust OD to zero
5. Pour the sample into a cuvette and place it inside
6. Take the readings as OD.

Calculation

$$\text{Concentration} = \frac{\text{OD of test} - \text{OD of blank}}{\text{OD of standard} - \text{OD of blank}} \times \text{Conc. of standard}$$

Care and Maintenance

1. Cover with a plastic cover
2. Keep the cuvette clean
3. Standardise the detector now and then

Differences between colorimeter and spectrophotometer		
S. No	*Colorimeter*	*Spectrophotometer*
1	Tungsten lamp for visible light	Halogen lamp for UV light
2	Filter is used	Prism or diffraction grating is used
3	Glass cuvette is used	Quartz cuvette is used
4	Visible wavelength is only available	UV and infrared wavelengths are also available
5	Band spectrum of wavelength over a wide range	Linear spectrum of wavelength over a narrow range
6	Less sensitive and less accurate	More sensitive and accurate
7	Less expensive	More expensive

CHAPTER

7

Autoanalysers

AUTOMATION

The process by which an instrument performs many tests with minimal involvement of analysts.

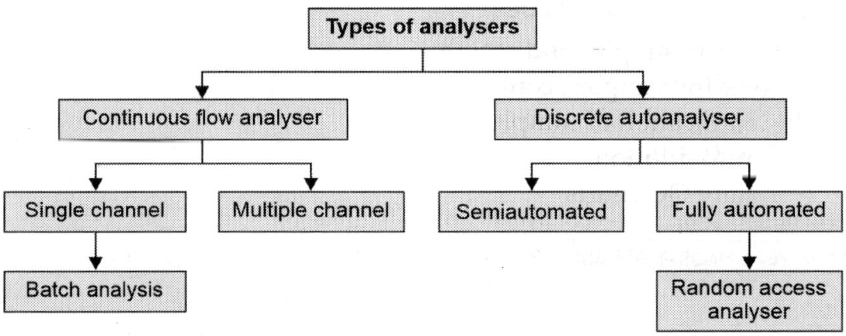

Continuous Flow Analyser

In this analyser, samples and reagents are passed continuously through the same stream. Individual samples are separated by air bubbles.

Single Channel Continuous Flow Analyser

Performs one parameter at a time

Multiple Channel Continuous Flow Analyser

Performs 6 or 12 parameters at a time

Disadvantages

1. Occupies large space in the lab
2. Performs a limited number of tests

DISCRETE ANALYSERS

1. It has a separate container for sample, reagent and reaction
2. It can run multiple tests on one sample or multiple samples for one test at a time

SEMIAUTOMATED ANALYSERS

1. Needs manual pipetting of reagent and sample and mixing
2. Performs reading of assays, displays test results, printing and storage of data

Disadvantages

1. More time consuming
2. More sample is needed
3. More chances of errors

FULLY AUTOMATED RANDOM ACCESS ANALYSERS

It can perform a variety of analytes for each specimen in batches. It has:

1. Automatic dispensing of reagents
2. Automatic dispensing of samples
3. Automatic mixing of reaction mixture
4. Different reagent packs

Special Features in Random Access Analysers

1. Level sensors for samples and reagents
2. Separate racks for samples, controls, calibrators
3. Bar code identification of samples and reagents
4. Facility for auto dilution
5. Plotting of daily QC charts

Example: Beckman Coulter AU 480, ERBA XL 640, Cobas e411 analyser

Advantages

1. More samples analysed in less time
2. More accuracy and precision of results
3. Less samples and reagents for each test
4. Less turnaround time (TAT).

CHAPTER

8

Electrophoresis

It is the movement of charged particles in an electric field

Principle

- Positively charged cations move towards the cathode
- Negatively charged anions move towards the anode.

Factors Affecting the Movement of Ions

1. Charge
2. Mass and shape
3. pH
4. Temperature

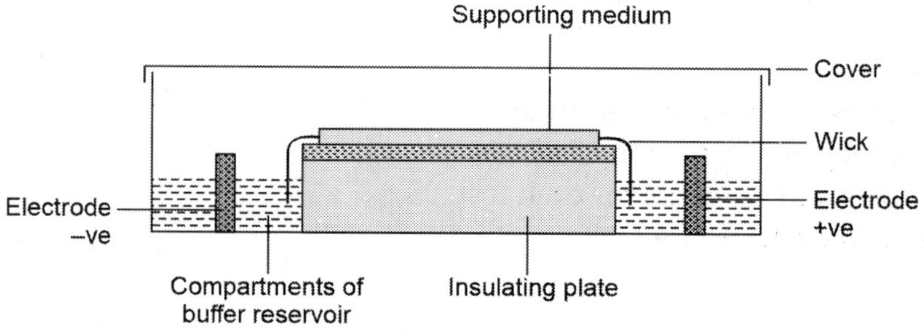

Electrophoresis apparatus

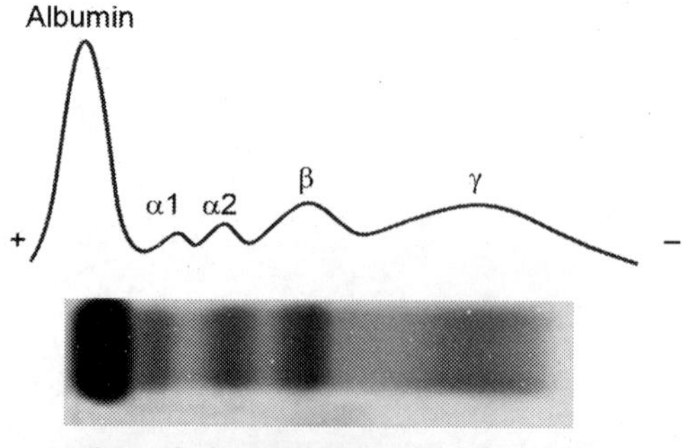

Separation of plasma proteins by electrophoresis

Types

1. Agarose gel electrophoresis
2. PAGE (polyacrylamide gel electrophoresis)
3. Capillary electrophoresis
4. Immunoelectrophoresis.

Applications

1. Diagnosis of multiple myeloma
2. Separation of serum proteins
3. Separation of CSF proteins
4. Separation of hemoglobin
5. Separation of lipoproteins.

Example: Automated Electophoresis—Sebia Hydragel.

CHAPTER

9

Chromatography

It is a technique for the separation of components of a mixture

Principle

1. Differential interaction of molecules between mobile phase and stationary phase
2. Molecules that interact with the mobile phase move faster
3. Molecules that interact with the stationary phase move slower

Types

1. Adsorption chromatography
2. Partition chromatography → Paper chromatography; → Thin layer chromatography
3. Gel filtration chromatography
4. Ion exchange chromatography
5. Gas-liquid chromatography
6. High-performance liquid chromatography (HPLC)
7. Affinity chromatography

$$R_f = \frac{\text{Distance traveled by solute}}{\text{Distance traveled by solvent}}$$

R_f values are used to identify each compound.

Applications

1. Separation of amino acids, carbohydrates, lipids
2. Diagnosis of amino acidurias
3. Separation of porphyrins
4. Separation and assay of vitamins, e.g. vitamin D
5. Separation and assay of haemoglobin, e.g. HbA1c by HPLC

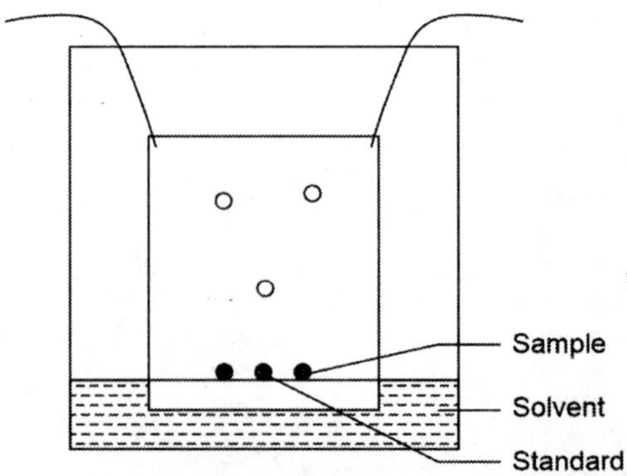

Thin layer chromatography

CHAPTER

10

Estimation of Electrolytes

ESTIMATION OF SODIUM

Methods

1. Ion selective electrode (ISE) method
2. Atomic absorption spectrometry (AAS)
3. Flame photometry

Normal level: 135–145 mmol/L

Hypernatremia

Serum sodium >155 mmol/L

Causes

1. Cushing's syndrome
2. Severe diarrhea
3. Diabetes insipidus

Hyponatremia

Serum sodium <130 mmol/L

Causes

1. SIADH
2. Heart failure
3. Chronic renal failure

ESTIMATION OF POTASSIUM

Methods

1. Ion selective electrode method (ISE)
2. Atomic absorption spectrometry (AAS)
3. Flame photometry

Normal level: 3.5–5 mmol/L

Hyperkalemia

Serum potassium > 5.5 mmol/L

Causes

1. Chronic renal failure
2. Addison's disease
3. Low insulin level

Hypokalemia

Serum potassium <3 mmol/L

1. Diarrhea
2. Vomiting
3. Insulin infusion

ESTIMATION OF CHLORIDE

Methods

1. Ion selective electrode method (ISE)
2. Titrimetric method (van slyke method)
3. Mercuric nitrate method–method of Schales and Schales

Normal level: 95–110 mmol/L

Causes of Decreased Levels of Chloride

1. Vomiting, diarrhea
2. Pyloric stenosis
3. Chronic renal failure
4. Diabetic coma

Causes of Increased Levels of Chloride

1. Renal tubular acidosis
2. Hyperparathyroidism

Samples for Estimation

1. Serum
2. Heparinized plasma
3. Sweat for chloride estimation
4. CSF
5. Urine

A hemolyzed sample is not suitable for electrolyte estimation. Samples are to be preserved at 2–8°C.

CHAPTER

11

Arterial Blood Gas (ABG) Analyser

INDICATIONS

1. To assess the blood pH
2. To diagnose acid–base disorders
3. For unconscious patients

Principle

Ion selective electrode (ISE) method

ISE Principle

The concentration of the ion is measured by difference in the electric potential by comparing it with a reference electrode.

Example:
1. pH electrode
2. Carbon electrode
3. Oxygen electrode
4. CO_2 electrode

Samples

1. Femoral artery
2. Brachial artery
3. Radial artery

Investigations

Measured Parameters

1. pH
2. pO_2
3. pCO_2

Calculated Parameters

4. HCO_3
5. Base excess
6. Anion gap

Uses

1. To measure blood gases and blood pH
2. To diagnose acid–base disorders:
   a. Metabolic acidosis
   b. Metabolic alkalosis
   c. Respiratory acidosis
   d. Respiratory alkalosis

Equipment

1. Radiometer ABL 80
2. Abbott i STAT

Indications to do ABG Testing

1. Critically ill patients
2. Patients with altered sensorium
3. Diagnosis of diabetic ketoacidosis (DKA)

CHAPTER

12

Enzyme-linked Immunosorbent Assay (ELISA)

ELISA: Enzyme-linked immunosorbent assay.

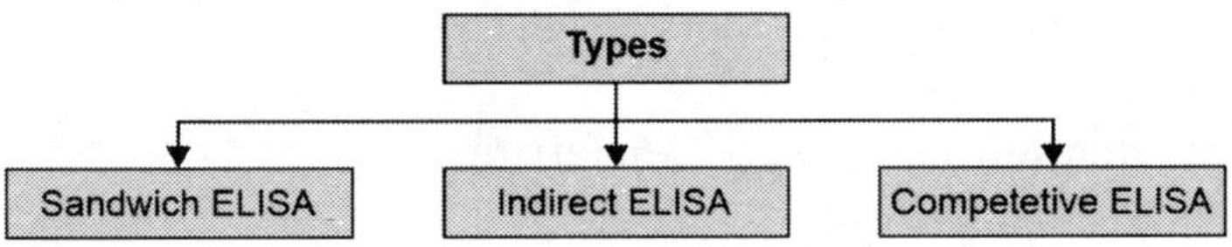

Reagents

1. Label enzymes
   - Alkaline phosphatase
   - Horseradish peroxidase
   - Glucose-6-phosphate dehydrogenase
2. Horseradish peroxidase
3. TMB substrate

Principle

Antigen is immobilized
↓
A detection antibody is added
↓
Forms an antigen-antibody complex
↓
Detection antibody is linked to an enzyme
↓
Enzyme gives colour to the addition of substrate
↓
Colour measures the quantity of antigen

Sandwich ELISA

1. "Capture Antibody" coated on a microtiter plate
2. Antigen in the sample binds to antibody
3. Secondary antibody binds to Ag-Ab complex
4. Secondary antibody is the detection antibody

Indirect ELISA

1. Antigen coated on a microtiter plate
2. Antibody to the antigen is added
3. Antibody is enzyme-linked

Example: HIV antibodies

Competitive ELISA

1. Antibodies coated on a microtiter plate
2. Sample antigen and standard antigen compete to bind the antibody

Example: T_3 and T_4 assay

Applications

1. Tumor markers assay, e.g. AFP, Beta HCG, CA 125
2. Thyroid function test, e.g. T_4, TSH
3. Inflammatory markers assay, e.g. IL-6, ferritin
4. Hormone assays, e.g. cortisol
5. Viral markers, e.g. HIV, HBsAg, HBV, HCV
6. RA factor

CHAPTER

13

Radioimmunoassay (RIA)

RIA, an assay utilizing radioisotopes. Commonly employs isotopes such as I^{125}, I^{131}, H^3 and Co^{57}.

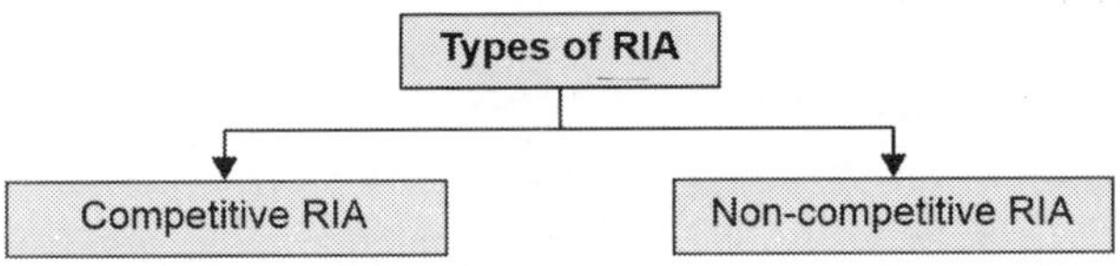

Competitive RIA

1. Competition between radiolabeled and unlabeled antigen/antibody
2. Concentration of tracer is inversely proportional to antigen measured
3. Can measure small quantities

Example: T_3, T_4 measurement

Non Competitive RIA

1. No competition
2. Two antibodies are capture antibody and signal antibody
3. Sandwich assay

Example: TSH, insulin assay

Applications of RIA

1. Hormones assay
2. Tumor markers assay
3. Thyroid function tests

Advantages of RIA

1. High sensitivity
2. High specificity

Disadvantages of RIA

1. Hazardous
2. Short shelf life of reagents

SECTION

III

Practical Biochemistry

1. Analysis of Normal Urine
2. Non-Protein Nitrogenous Substances (NPN)
3. Abnormal Constituents of Urine
4. Estimation of Plasma Glucose
5. Estimation of Serum Urea
6. Estimation of Serum Creatinine
7. Estimation of Serum Total Protein
8. Estimation of Serum Albumin
9. Estimation of Serum Total Cholesterol
10. Estimation of Serum Triglycerides
11. Estimation of Serum HDL Cholesterol
12. Estimation of Serum Bilirubin
13. Estimation of Serum SGOT/AST
14. Estimation of Serum SGPT/ALT
15. Estimation of Serum Calcium
16. Estimation of Serum Phosphorus
17. Estimation of Serum Amylase
18. Estimation of Serum Lipase
19. Estimation of Glucose by Standardisation
20. Estimation of Urea by Standardisation
21. Estimation of Creatinine by Standardisation
22. Test for Carbohydrates
23. Test for Proteins
24. Test for Lipids
25. OSPE Stations
26. *Viva Voce* Questions and Answers

CHAPTER

1

Analysis of Normal Urine

Urine is an ultrafiltrate of plasma that contains 95% water and dissolved solutes like Urea, creatinine, electrolytes, other organic and inorganic compounds. Urinalysis involves examining various physical properties and chemical constituents of urine:

S. No	*Experiment*	*Observation*	*Inference*
I. 1	**Physical examination** **Color**	Straw colored	Due to the presence of urochrome pigment
2	**Appearance**	Clear	Normal urine is clear and transparent
3	**pH**	pH of the given urine is 6.8	pH of normal urine is 4.6 to 8
4	**Specific gravity** Fill 3/4th of the glass cylinder with urine. The urinometer is allowed to float in the cylinder without touching the sides. Note the marking graduated on the stem of the urinometer at the level of the upper surface of urine	The specific gravity of the given urine sample is 1.020	The normal specific gravity of urine ranges from 1.003 to 1.030
II A 1.	**Chemical reactions** **Inorganic constituents** **Test for chloride** To 3 ml of urine in a test tube, add 0.5 ml of concentrated nitric acid. Mix and add 1 ml of 3% silver nitrate solution	A white precipitate is formed	Presence of chloride (formation of a white precipitate of silver chloride)
2.	**Test for calcium** Take 2 ml of urine in a test tube, add 2 ml of 2% potassium oxalate solution	A white precipitate is formed	Presence of calcium (formation of a white precipitate of calcium oxalate)
3.	**Test for inorganic sulphates** To 5 ml of urine in a test tube add 1 ml of conc. HCl. Mix well and add 5 ml of 10% barium chloride solution	A white precipitate is formed	Presence of inorganic sulphates in urine (formation of a white precipitate of barium sulphate)
B 1.	**Organic constituents** **Test for ethereal sulphates** Filter off the precipitate obtained in the above experiment. Boil the filtrate	A white precipitate is formed	Presence of inorganic sulphates in urine (formation of a white precipitate of barium sulphate)

Result

The inorganic constituents in normal urine are chloride, calcium and inorganic sulphates. The organic constituents are ethereal sulphates and non-protein nitrogenous substances.

CHAPTER

2

Non-Protein Nitrogenous Substances

Non-protein nitrogenous substances (NPN) encompass a diverse array of compounds in biological systems that contain nitrogen but are not proteins. NPN of clinical significance include urea, creatinine and uric acid. These are used as biomarkers of renal function and are normal constituents of urine.

- Urea is the end product of protein breakdown.
- Creatinine is a muscle protein.
- Uric acid is the end product of purine breakdown.
- The following are the qualitative tests to detect NPN in urine.

S. No	*Experiment*	*Observation*	*Inference*
1.	**Specific urease test for urea** To 3 ml of sample in a test tube, add a pinch of horse gram powder. Mix well and add a drop of phenolphthalein indicator	A pink color solution is formed	Presence of urea (urease in horsegram powder breakdown urea to liberate ammonia that turns phenolphthalein indicator pink)
2.	**Benedict's uric acid test for uric acid** To 3 ml of sample in a test tube, add 1 ml of Benedict's uric acid reagent and 1 ml of 20% sodium carbonate and mix	A dark blue color solution is formed	Presence of uric acid (uric acid is a reducing agent that reduces phosphotungstic acid to tungsten blue)
3.	**Schiff's test for uric acid** Wet the filter paper with a few drops of ammoniacal silver nitrate. Add 2 to 3 drops of sample on the paper	A black color is formed on the filter paper	Presence of uric acid (uric acid is a reducing agent that reduces ammonical silver nitrate to metallic silver)
4.	**Jaffe's test for creatinine** Take 3 ml of sample in a test tube and 3 ml of distilled water in a control tube. In both the tubes, add 1 ml of picric acid and 10 drops of 10% NaOH. Mix well	Test tube—reddish-orange color is formed control tube—yellow color is formed	Presence of creatinine (Creatinine reacts with picric acid in alkaline medium to form creatinine picrate)

Result

The non-protein nitrogenous substances are urea, uric acid and creatinine.

CHAPTER

3

Abnormal Constituents of Urine

The abnormal constituents that may be found in urine are:

1. Reducing sugars
2. Ketone bodies
3. Proteins
4. Blood
5. Bile salts
6. Bile pigments

TEST FOR REDUCING SUGARS

Benedict's Test

Principle: Sugars form enediols in an alkaline medium that reduces cupric ions (Cu^{++}) of copper sulfate to cuprous ions (Cu^{+}) that form cuprous oxide that is red in color. Benedict's test is a semiquantitative test since the color of cuprous oxide depends on the amount of reducing substance in urine.

Colour	*Concentration of reducing substance in urine*	*Qualitative result*
Blue	Absence of reducing sugar	Negative
Green	< 0.5 g%	+
Yellow	1–1.5 g%	++
Orange	1.5–2 g%	+++
Red	>2 g%	++++

Non-carbohydrate reducing substances that may give a positive Benedict's test are:

1. Vitamin C
2. Homogentisic acid
3. Salicylates
4. Uric acid
5. Creatinine

TEST FOR KETONE BODIES

Principle of Rothera's Test

Ketone bodies (acetone and acetoacetate) react with sodium nitroprusside in an alkaline medium to form a purple color complex.

TEST FOR PROTEINS

1. Heat coagulation test
2. Heller's test
3. Sulfosalicylic acid test

Principle of Heat Coagulation Test

Heat causes denaturation of proteins by removing the shell of hydration and precipitates them.

Principle of Heller's Test

Acids cause denaturation of proteins by removing the shell of hydration and precipitates them.

Principle of Sulfosalicylic Acid Test

Sulfosalicylic acid is an alkaloid that causes the denaturation of proteins by removing the shell of hydration and neutralize their charge and precipitates them.

TEST FOR BLOOD

Principle of Benzidine Test

Heme has peroxidase activity that converts H_2O_2 to H_2O and nascent oxygen. Nascent oxygen combines with benzidine to form a blue-colored complex.

TEST FOR BILE SALTS

Principle of Hay's Test

Bile salts act as surfactants which reduce the surface tension. So the sulfur powder sinks to the bottom of the tube.
Bile salts are sodium taurocholate and sodium taurochenodeoxycholate.

TEST FOR BILE PIGMENTS

Principle of Fouchet's Test

$MgSO_4$ and $BaCl_2$ form $BaSO_4$ precipitate that adsorbs bilirubin. $FeCl_3$ in Fouchet's reagent oxidizes bilirubin to biliverdin which is green in color. Bile pigments are bilirubin and biliverdin.

Experiment	*Observation*	*Inference*
Test for reducing sugars **Benedict's test:** Take 5 ml of Benedict's reagent in a test tube and test for autoreduction by heating it. Add 8 drops of urine. Mix well and boil for 2 mins. Allow to cool	Brick red precipitate	Presence of reducing sugars (Glucose, Fructose)

Contd...

Experiment	*Observation*	*Inference*
Test for ketone bodies **Rothera's test:** Take 5 ml of urine in a test tube and saturate it with ammonium sulfate. Add 2 drops of 2% sodium nitroprusside. Mix well and add 1 ml of liquor ammonia along the sides of the tube	Purple color ring is formed at the junction of two liquids	Presence of ketone bodies
Test for proteins **Heat coagulation test:** Fill 3/4th of the test tube with urine and heat the upper 1/3rd of the tube while the lower 2/3rd serves as a control. Add 2–3 drops of 1% acetic acid	A white coagulum is formed Coagulum remains	Presence of proteins
Heller's test: Take 5 ml of urine in a test tube. Add 1 ml of conc. HNO_3 along the sides of the test tube	A white ring is formed at the junction of two liquids	Presence of proteins
Sulfosalicylic acid test: Take 3 ml of urine in a test tube. Add 2–3 drops of sulfosalicylic acid	White precipitate is formed	Presence of proteins
Test for blood **Benzidine test:** Take 1 ml of glacial acetic acid in a test tube and add a knife point of benzidine powder and dissolve. Add 1 ml of hydrogen peroxide and 1 ml of preheated urine in a test tube	A transient blue-green color turns to black is formed.	Presence of blood
Test for Bile salts **Hay's test:** Take 3 ml of urine in a test tube and 3 ml of water in a control tube. Sprinkle a pinch of sulphur powder over both the test tubes	Test tube—sulphur powder sinks Control tube—sulphur powder floats	Presence of bile salts
Test for bile pigments **Fouchet's test:** To 3 ml of urine in a test tube, add magnesium sulphate crystals, mix well and add 2 ml of 10% barium chloride. A white precipitate is formed. Filter the precipitate using filter paper. Allow it to dry and add 1–2 drops of Fouchet's reagent over it	A green color develops on the filter paper	Presence of bile pigments

Result

The abnormal constituents of urine in the given sample are ________________ and ________________.

CHAPTER

4

Estimation of Plasma Glucose

Aim: To estimate the concentration of glucose in the given sample by glucose oxidase peroxidase method

Method: Glucose oxidase peroxidase (GOD–POD) method

Principle

Glucose present in plasma is oxidized to gluconic acid and hydrogen peroxide by glucose oxidase. Hydrogen peroxide is then converted to water and oxygen by peroxidase. 4-Amino antipyrine accepts oxygen with phenol to give a pink chromogen. The color intensity is directly proportional to glucose concentration measured at 540 nm (green filter) using a colorimeter.

Procedure

Label 3 test tubes as blank (B), standard (S) and test (T)

S. No.	*Reagents*	*Blank*	*Standard*	*Test*
1	Distilled water	10 µl	–	–
2	Glucose standard	–	10 µl	–
3	Test	–	–	10 µl
4	Glucose oxidase (GOD) and peroxidase (POD) reagent	1 ml	1 ml	1 ml

Mix well and keep at room temperature for 10 minutes.
Measure optical densities (OD) at 540 nm.

Calculation

$$\text{Concentration of glucose} = \frac{\text{OD of test} - \text{OD of blank}}{\text{OD of standard} - \text{OD of blank}} \times \text{Conc. of standard}$$

$$= \frac{\text{T} - \text{B}}{\text{S} - \text{B}} \times 100 \text{ mg/dL}$$

$$= \underline{\qquad\qquad} \text{ mg/dL}$$

Result

The concentration of glucose in the given sample of plasma is _______ mg/dL.

Clinical Significance

Reference Range

Fasting blood glucose 70 to 100 mg/dL
Postprandial blood glucose <140 mg/dL
Random blood glucose <140 mg/dL

Causes of Hypoglycemia

1. Hyperinsulinemia
2. Liver disorders
3. Starvation
4. von Gierke's disease

Causes of Hyperglycemia

1. Diabetes mellitus
2. Cushing's syndrome
3. Hyperthyroidism

Other Methods

1. Copper reduction method
2. Nelson-Somogyi method
3. Asatoor and King method
4. Folin-Wu method

Enzymatic Method

1. Hexokinase method
2. Glucokinase method.

CHAPTER

5

Estimation of Serum Urea

Aim: To estimate the concentration of urea in the given serum sample by diacetyl monoxime method.

Method: Diacetyl monoxime–thiosemicarbazide (DAM–TSC) method.

Principle

Urea present in the sample reacts with diacetyl monoxime in the hot acidic medium in the presence of ferric chloride to give a pink-colored complex. Thiosemicarbazide acts as a catalyst. The color intensity is directly proportional to the concentration of urea measured at 540 nm (green filter) using a colorimeter.

Procedure

Label 3 test tubes as blank (B), standard (S) and test (T)

S. No.	*Reagents*	*Blank*	*Standard*	*Test*
1	Distilled water	20 µl	–	–
2	Standard	–	20 µl	–
3	Test	–	–	20 µl
4	Diacetyl monoxime/ thiosemicarbazide	1.5 ml	1.5 ml	1.5 ml
5	Acid mixture	1.5 ml	1.5 ml	1.5 ml

Mix well and incubate in a water bath for 20 minutes. Cool it. Measure optical densities (OD) at 540 nm.

Calculation

$$\text{Concentration of urea} = \frac{\text{OD of test} - \text{OD of blank}}{\text{OD of standard} - \text{OD of blank}} \times \text{Conc. of standard}$$

$$= \frac{T - B}{S - B} \times 50 \text{ mg/dL}$$

$$= \_\_\_\_\_\_\_\_\_\_ \text{ mg/dL}$$

Result

The concentration of urea in the given sample of serum is ______________ mg/dL.

Clinical Significance

Reference Range

Normal level of urea in blood = 15 to 35 mg/dL.

Causes of Increased Blood Urea (Uremia)

Prerenal Causes

1. Burns
2. Hemorrhage
3. Shock

Renal Causes

1. Acute glomerulonephritis
2. Renal failure
3. Malignant hypertension

Postrenal Causes

1. Enlarged prostate
2. Stricture urethra
3. Urinary tract stones
4. Tumours of the urinary bladder

Causes for Decreased Blood Urea

1. Low protein diet
2. Severe liver disease
3. Overhydration

Other Methods

1. Nesslerization method
2. **Enzymatic method:** Glutamate dehydrogenase-urease method.

CHAPTER

6

Estimation of Serum Creatinine

Aim: To estimate the concentration of creatinine in the given serum sample by Jaffe's method

Method: Alkaline picrate method (Jaffe's method)

Principle

Creatinine in the sample reacts with picric acid in an alkaline medium to form red orange-colored compound creatinine picrate. The color intensity is directly proportional to the creatinine concentration in the sample which is measured at 490 nm using a blue filter.

Procedure

Label 3 test tubes as blank (B), standard (S) and test (T)

S. No.	*Reagents*	*Blank*	*Standard*	*Test*
1	Distilled water	200 µl	–	–
2	Standard	–	200 µl	–
3	Test	–	–	200 µl
4	NaOH	1 ml	1 ml	1 ml
5	Picric acid	1 ml	1 ml	1 ml

Mix well and incubate for 10 minutes at room temperature.
Measure optical densities (OD) at 490 nm.

Calculation

$$\text{Concentration of creatinine} = \frac{\text{OD of test} - \text{OD of blank}}{\text{OD of standard} - \text{OD of blank}} \times \text{Conc. of standard}$$

$$= \frac{T - B}{S - B} \times 2 \text{ mg/dL}$$

= ___________ mg/dL

Result

The concentration of creatinine in the given sample of serum is __________ mg/dL.

Clinical Significance

Reference Range

Normal serum creatinine = 0.6–1.2 mg/dL (females)
0.7–1.4 mg/dL (males)

Normal creatinine excretion in urine = 1.5 to 2.5 g/day

Causes of Increased Serum Creatinine

Prerenal Cause

1. Dehydration
2. Shock

Renal Cause

1. Renal failure
2. Acute glomerulonephritis

Postrenal Cause

1. Bladder cancer
2. Urinary tract stones

Other Methods of Creatinine Estimation

1. Enzymatic method
2. Creatinase method
3. Creatininase method

CHAPTER

7

Estimation of Serum Total Protein

Aim: To estimate the concentration of total protein in the given serum sample.

Method: Biuret method (colorimetric method).

Principle

Proteins with two or more peptide bonds react with copper sulphate in biuret reagent in alkaline medium and form a coordination complex with the nitrogen of peptide bond. This complex is purple in color.

The color intensity is directly proportional to protein concentration measured at 540 nm (green filter) using a colorimeter.

Procedure

Label 3 test tubes as Blank (B), Standard (S) and Test (T)

S. No.	*Reagents*	*B*	*S*	*T*
1	Distilled water	0.1 ml	–	–
2	Protein standard (6 g/dL)	–	0.1 ml	–
3	Test	–	–	0.1 ml
4	Biuret reagent	2 ml	2 ml	2 ml

Mix well and wait at room temperature for 20 minutes.
Measure optical densities (OD) at 540 nm.

Calculation

$$\text{Concentration of total protein} = \frac{\text{OD of test} - \text{OD of blank}}{\text{OD of standard} - \text{OD of blank}} \times \text{Conc. of standard}$$

$$= \frac{\text{T} - \text{B}}{\text{S} - \text{B}} \times 6 \text{ g/dL}$$

$$= \_\_\_\_\_\_\_\_\_\_ \text{ g/dL}$$

Result

The concentration of total protein in the given sample of serum is __________ g/dL.

Clinical Significance

Reference range: 6 to 8 gm/dL.

Increased total protein concentration is seen in:

- Hemoconcentration
- Dehydration
- Vomiting
- Diarrhea
- Tuberculosis
- Multiple myeloma

Decreased total protein concentration is seen in:

- Malnutrition
- Liver disease
- Nephrotic syndrome
- Cancer
- Pregnancy

Normal albumin–globulin ratio is 1.2 to 1.5:1.

Reversal of the albumin–globulin ratio is seen in nephrotic syndrome and chronic infections.

Other Methods of Total Protein Estimation

1. Lowry's method
2. Kjeldahl—nesslerization method
3. Copper sulphate specific gravity method

CHAPTER

8

Estimation of Serum Albumin

Aim: To estimate the concentration of albumin in the given serum sample.

Method: BCG method (bromocresol green method).

Principle

At pH 4.2, albumin reacts with BCG and gives a blue-green color. The color intensity is directly proportional to albumin concentration that is measured at 630 nm using a colorimeter.

Procedure

Label 3 test tubes as blank (B), standard (S) and test (T)

S. No.	*Reagents*	*B*	*S*	*T*
1	Distilled water	10 μl	–	–
2	Standard	–	10 μl	–
3	Test	–	–	10 μl
4	Albumin reagent	1000 μl	1000 μl	1000 μl

Mix well. Measure optical densities (OD) at 630 nm after 1 min incubation at 37°C.

Calculation

$$\text{Concentration of serum albumin} = \frac{\text{OD of test} - \text{OD of blank}}{\text{OD of standard} - \text{OD of blank}} \times \text{Conc. of standard}$$

$$= \frac{T - B}{S - B} \times 3.6 \text{ g/dL}$$

= __________ g/dL

Result

The concentration of albumin in the given sample of serum is __________ g/dL.

Clinical Significance

Reference range
Serum albumin= 3.5 to 5 g/dL
Serum globulin = Total protein–albumin

Increased albumin concentration is seen in:

- Dehydration

Decreased albumin concentration is seen in:

- Malnutrition
- Liver disease
- Nephrotic syndrome

Normal albumin–globulin ratio is 1.2 to 1.5:1.

Reversal of the albumin–globulin ratio is seen in nephrotic syndrome and chronic infections.

Other Methods of Albumin Estimation

1. Turbidimetry
2. Esbach's albuminometer.

CHAPTER

9

Estimation of Serum Total Cholesterol

Aim: To estimate the concentration of total cholesterol in the given serum sample.

Method: Cholesterol oxidase peroxidase method.

Principle

$$\text{Cholesterol ester} + H_2O \xrightarrow{\text{Cholesterol esterase}} \text{Cholesterol} + \text{fatty acids}$$

$$\text{Cholesterol} + O_2 \xrightarrow{\text{Cholesterol oxidase}} \text{Cholestenone} + H_2O_2$$

$$2H_2O_2 + 4AAP + \text{Phenol} \xrightarrow{\text{Peroxidase}} \text{Quinoneimine dye} + 4H_2O$$

The absorbance of quinoneimine so formed is directly proportional to the cholesterol concentration at 505 nm.

Procedure

Take 3 test tubes and label them as blank (B), standard (S) and test (T)

S. No.	*Reagents*	*B*	*S*	*T*
1	Distilled water	10 μl	–	–
2	Standard	–	10 μl	–
3	Test	–	–	10 μl
4	Working reagent	1000 μl	1000 μl	1000 μl

Mix well, incubate at 37°C for 10 minutes and read the absorbance using a semi-autoanalyzer

Calculation

$$\text{Concentration of cholesterol} = \frac{\text{Absorbance of test}}{\text{Absorbance of standard}} \times \text{Conc. of standard}$$

$$= \frac{T}{S} \times 200$$

$$= \_\_\_\_\_\_\_\_\_\_ \text{ mg/dL}$$

Result

The concentration of cholesterol in the given sample of serum is ________ mg/dL.

Clinical Significance

Reference range

Desirable	≤200 mg/dL
Borderline high	200–239 mg/dL
High	≥240 mg/dL

Causes of Hypercholesterolemia

1. Nephrotic syndrome
2. Diabetes mellitus
3. Atherosclerosis
4. Obstructive jaundice
5. Myxoedema
6. Obesity
7. Cirrhosis
8. Xanthomatosis

Causes of Hypocholesterolemia

1. Malabsorption syndrome
2. Hyperthyroidism
3. Statins therapy
4. Pernicious anemia
5. Hemolytic jaundice

Other Methods of Cholesterol Estimation

1. Colorimetric method (Zak's method).

CHAPTER

10

Estimation of Serum Triglycerides

Aim: To estimate the concentration of triglycerides in the given serum sample.

Method: GPO PAP method

Principle

$$\text{Triglycerides} + H_2O \xrightarrow{\text{LPL}} \text{Glycerol} + \text{Free fattyacids}$$

$$\text{Glycerol + ATP} \xrightarrow{\text{GK}} \text{Glycerol-3-phosphate + ADP}$$

$$\text{Glycerol-3-phosphate} + O_2 \xrightarrow{\text{GPO}} \text{DAP} + H_2O_2$$

$$H_2O_2 + \text{4AAP} + \text{4-Chlorophenol} \xrightarrow{\text{POD}} \text{Quinoneimine} + H_2O$$

The absorbance of quinoneimine is directly proportional to the triglyceride concentration at 546 nm.

Procedure

Label 3 test tubes as blank (B), standard (S) and test (T)

S. No.	*Reagents*	*B*	*S*	*T*
1	Distilled water	10 µl	–	–
2	Standard	–	10 µl	–
3	Test	–	–	10 µl
4	Working reagent	1000 µl	1000 µl	1000 µl

Mix well and incubate for 5 minutes at 37°C. Read the absorbance using a semi-autoanalyzer.

Calculation

$$\text{Concentration of triglyceride} = \frac{\text{Absorbance of test}}{\text{Absorbance of standard}} \times \text{Conc. of standard}$$

$$= \frac{T}{S} \times \text{Conc. of standard}$$

$$= \_\_\_\_\_\_\_\_\_\_ \text{ mg/dL}$$

Result

The concentration of triglyceride in the given sample of serum is _________ mg/dL.

Clinical Significance

Reference range: 50–150 mg/dL

Causes of Hypertriglyceridemia

1. Hypothyroidism
2. Nephrotic syndrome
3. Diabetes mellitus
4. Metabolic syndrome

Causes of Hypotriglyceridemia

1. Hyperthyroidism
2. Malnutrition.

CHAPTER

11

Estimation of Serum HDL Cholesterol

Aim: To estimate the HDL cholesterol concentration in the given serum sample.

Method 1: Enzymatic method by precipitation.

Principle

The apo-B-containing lipoproteins (chylomicrons, LDL, IDL and VLDL) are precipitated using phosphotungstic acid in the presence of magnesium. The supernatant contains HDL cholesterol which is estimated by the cholesterol oxidase-peroxidase method.

Method 2: Direct HDL estimation.

Principle

Binding agents bind to apo-B-containing lipoproteins and block them from the action of cholesterol oxidase. HDL cholesterol alone participates in the reaction catalysed by cholesterol oxidase—peroxidase which is then estimated. This homogenous assay does not require precipitation and manual separation, hence suitable for automation.

Clinical Significance

Reference range:

Males: 40–70 mg/dL
Females: 50–80 mg/dL

ATP-III Classification

HDL cholesterol <40—Low
≥60—High

Low Levels of HDL Cholesterol

Increased risk of atherosclerosis and coronary artery disease.

Low levels of HDL cholesterol is seen in hypoalphalipoproteinemia (Tangier's disease)

LDL Cholesterol Calculation

LDL cholesterol is calculated using Friedewald formula when the triglyceride concentration is $\leq$400 mg/dL.

$$\text{LDL cholesterol} = \text{Total cholesterol} - (\text{HDL} + \text{VLDL})$$

$$\text{VLDL cholesterol} = \frac{\text{Triglyceride}}{5}$$

CHAPTER

12

Estimation of Serum Bilirubin

Aim: To estimate the concentration of bilirubin in the given serum sample.

Method: Diazo method (Malloy–Evelyn method).

Principle

Diazo's method is based on the van den Bergh reaction. Bilirubin in the sample reacts with diazotized sulfanilic acid to form reddish-purple azobilirubin. The color intensity is directly proportional to bilirubin concentration measured at 560 nm using a semi-autoanalyser.

Procedure

Label 3 test tubes as blank (B), standard (S) and test (T)

S. No.	*Reagents*	*B*	*S*	*T*
1	Distilled water	50 µl	–	–
2	Standard	–	50 µl	–
3	Test	–	–	50 µl
4	Reagent	1000 µl	1000 µl	1000 µl

Mix well and incubate at 37°C for 5 minutes.
Measure optical densities (OD) at 540 nm.

Calculation

$$\text{The concentration of bilirubin} = \frac{\text{OD of test} - \text{OD of blank}}{\text{OD of standard} - \text{OD of blank}} \times \text{Conc. of standard}$$

$$= \frac{\text{T} - \text{B}}{\text{S} - \text{B}} \times \text{Conc. of standard}$$

$$= \_\_\_\_\_\_\_\_\_\_ \text{ mg/dL}$$

Result

The concentration of bilirubin in the given serum sample is ________________ mg/dL.

Clinical Significance

Reference range: Total bilirubin: 0.2 to 1 mg/dL
Direct bilirubin: 0 to 0.2 mg/dL

Clinical condition: Jaundice

Types of Jaundice

As per the site of action:

1. Prehepatic jaundice
2. Hepatic jaundice
3. Posthepatic jaundice

As per the pathological cause:

1. Hemolytic jaundice
2. Hepatocellular jaundice
3. Obstructive jaundice

As per bilirubin:

1. Conjugated hyperbilirubinemia
2. Unconjugated hyperbilirubinemia

Causes of hemolytic jaundice:

1. Incompatible blood transfusion
2. Rh incompatibility
3. Hemolytic anemia

Causes of hepatocellular jaundice:

1. Viral hepatitis
2. Alcoholic hepatitis
3. NAFLD

Causes of obstructive jaundice:

1. Gallstones
2. Biliary strictures
3. Carcinoma of head of pancreas.

CHAPTER

13

Estimation of Serum SGOT/AST

Aim: To estimate the enzymatic activity of SGOT/AST (serum glutamate oxaloacetate transferase/aspartate transaminase) in the given serum sample.

Method: International Federation of Clinical Chemistry (IFCC) method.

Principle

$$\text{Aspartate} + \text{Alpha ketoglutarate} \xrightarrow{\text{AST/SGOT}} \text{Oxalacetate} + \text{Glutamate}$$

$$\text{Oxaloacetate} + \text{NADH} \xrightarrow{\text{Malate dehydrogenase}} \text{Malate} + \text{NAD}^{+}$$

The rate of decrease in absorbance of NADH at 340 nm is directly proportional to the enzymatic activity of SGOT (AST), which is measured using a semi-autoanalyser.

Procedure

Take 3 test tubes and label them as blank (B), standard (S) and test (T). No incubation is needed. The absorbance is measured in a semi-autoanalyser.

S. No.	*Reagents*	*B*	*S*	*T*
1	Distilled water	50 µl	–	–
2	Standard	–	50 µl	–
3	Test	–	–	50 µl
4	Working reagent	500 µl	500 µl	500 µl

Calculation

$$\text{Enzymatic activity of SGOT} = \frac{\text{Absorbance of test}}{\text{Absorbance of standard}} \times \text{Conc. of standard}$$

$$= \_\_\_\_\_\_\_\_\_\_ \text{IU/L}$$

Result

The enzymatic activity of SGOT in the given serum sample is __________ IU/L.

Clinical Significance

Reference range: 5 to 35 IU/L

Causes of Increased SGOT

1. Hepatitis
2. Cirrhosis
3. Pancreatitis
4. Myocardial infarction
5. Chronic alcoholism

Causes of Decreased SGOT

1. Anemia
2. Vitamin B_6 deficiency
3. Drugs like metronidazole

Other Methods of SGOT Estimation

1. DNPH method.

CHAPTER

14

Estimation of Serum SGPT/ALT

Aim: To estimate the enzymatic activity of SGPT/ALT (serum glutamate pyruvate transaminase/alanine transaminase) in the given serum sample.

Method: International Federation of Clinical Chemistry (IFCC) method

Principle

The rate of decrease in NADH absorbance at 340 nm is directly proportional to the enzymatic activity of SGPT (ALT) that is measured using a semi-autoanalyser.

Procedure

$$\text{Alanine} + \text{alpha ketoglutarate} \xrightarrow{\text{ALT/SGPT}} \text{Pyruvate} + \text{glutamate}$$

$$\text{Pyruvate} + \text{NADH} \xrightarrow{\text{Lactate dehydrogenase}} \text{Lactate} + \text{NAD}^+$$

Label 3 test tubes as blank (B), standard (S) and test (T). Incubation is not required. The absorbance is measured in a semi-autoanalyser.

S. No.	*Reagents*	*B*	*S*	*T*
1	Distilled water	50 μl	–	–
2	Standard	–	50 μl	–
3	Test	–	–	50 μl
4	Working reagent	500 μl	500 μl	500 μl

Calculation

$$\text{Enzymatic activity of SGPT} = \frac{\text{Absorbance of test}}{\text{Absorbance of standard}} \times \text{Conc. of standard}$$

$$= \_\_\_\_\_\_\_\_\_\_\_\_ \text{ IU/L}$$

Result

The enzymatic activity of SGPT in the given serum sample is ____________ IU/L.

Clinical Significance

Reference range:

Males: 13 to 35 IU/L
Females: 10 to 30 IU/L

Causes of Increased SGPT

1. Hepatitis
2. Cirrhosis
3. Hepatocellular carcinoma

Causes of Decreased SGPT

1. Vitamin B_6 deficiency
2. Chronic kidney disease

Other Methods of SGPT Estimation

1. DNPH method.

CHAPTER

15

Estimation of Serum Calcium

Aim: To estimate the concentration of total calcium in the given serum sample.

Method: Arsenazo method

Principle

At pH 6.75, calcium ions react with arsenazo to form colored chromophores. The absorbance is measured at 650 nm and is proportional to the concentration of calcium.

Procedure

Label 3 test tubes as blank (B), standard (S) and test (T)

S. No.	*Reagents*	*B*	*S*	*T*
1	Distilled water	20 µl	–	–
2	Standard	–	20 µl	–
3	Test	–	–	20 µl
4	Working reagent	1000 µl	1000 µl	1000 µl

Mix well and measure Optical densities (OD) at 650 nm.

Calculation

$$\text{The concentration of calcium} = \frac{\text{OD of test}}{\text{OD of standard}} \times \text{Conc. of standard}$$

$$= \frac{T}{S} \times 10$$

$$= \_\_\_\_\_\_\_\_\_\_ \text{ mg/dL}$$

Result

The concentration of total calcium in the given serum sample is __________ mg/dL.

Clinical Significance

Reference range: 9 to 11 mg/dL

Causes of Hypercalcemia

1. Hyperparathyroidism
2. Bone metastasis
3. Paget's disease
4. Thyrotoxicosis
5. Benign familial hypercalcemia
6. Multiple myeloma

Causes of Hypocalcemia

1. Vitamin D deficiency
2. Parathyroid hormone deficiency
3. Increased calcitonin (medullary carcinoma of the thyroid)
4. Acute pancreatitis
5. Intestinal malabsorption
6. Hypoalbuminemia

Other Methods of Calcium Estimation

1. O-cresolphthalein method
2. Clark and Collip method.

CHAPTER

16

Estimation of Serum Phosphorus

Aim: To estimate the concentration of phosphorus in the given serum sample.

Method: Endpoint method using ammonium molybdate.

Principle

Inorganic phosphate reacts with ammonium molybdate in the presence of sulphuric acid to form ammonium phosphomolybdate complex. The amount of phosphomolybdate formed is directly proportional to the concentration of inorganic phosphate.

$$\text{Phosphate + Ammonium molybdate} \xrightarrow{H_2SO_4} \text{ammonium phosphomolybdate}$$

Procedure

Label 3 test tubes as blank (B), standard (S) and test (T)

S. No.	*Reagents*	*B*	*S*	*T*
1	Distilled water	20 μl	–	–
2	Standard	–	20 μl	–
3	Test	–	–	20 μl
4	Working reagent	1000 μl	1000 μl	1000 μl

Mix well, wait for 10 minutes and measure optical densities (OD) at 340 nm.

Calculation

$$\text{Concentration of phosphorus} = \frac{\text{OD of test} - \text{OD of blank}}{\text{OD of standard} - \text{OD of blank}} \times \text{Conc. of standard}$$

$$= \frac{T - B}{S - B} \times 5$$

$$= \_\_\_\_\_\_\_\_\_\_ \text{ mg/dL}$$

Result

The concentration of phosphorus in the given serum sample is __________ mg/dL.

Clinical Significance

Reference range:

Adults: 3 to 4 mg/dL
Children: 5 to 6 mg/dL

Causes of Hyperphosphatemia

1. Increased phosphate absorption
2. Decreased excretion of phosphate
   - Renal impairment
3. Increased cell lysis
   - Bone metastasis
   - Cancer chemotherapy
4. Hypocalcemia
5. Hypoparathyroidism

Causes of Hypophosphatemia

1. Decreased phosphate absorption
2. Respiratory alkalosis
3. Hyperparathyroidism
4. Hypercalcemia
5. Hereditary hypophosphatemia

Other Methods of Phosphorus Estimation

- Fiske-Subbarow method.

CHAPTER

17

Estimation of Serum Amylase

Aim: To estimate the concentration of amylase in the given serum sample.

Method: CNP-G3 method.

Principle

$$\text{Gal-G2-}\alpha\text{CNP} \xrightarrow{\text{Amylase}} \text{Gal-G2} + \text{CNP}$$

$$\text{CNP-G3} \rightarrow \text{2-chloro-4-nitrophenol-}\alpha\text{-maltotrioside}$$

This is a direct assay. Does not require alpha-glucosidase activity. The rate of CNP formation measured at 415 nm is proportional to alpha-amylase activity.

Procedure

- **Sample volume:** 4 µl
- **R1 volume:** 200 µl
- **Primary wavelength:** 415 nm
- **Secondary wavelength:** 700 nm
- **Assay type:** Kinetic assay
- **Curve type:** Linear increasing slope
- **Linearity:** 10 to 1500 U/L

Calculation

$$\text{The concentration of amylase} = \frac{\text{OD of test} - \text{OD of blank}}{\text{OD of standard} - \text{OD of blank}} \times \text{Conc. of standard}$$

Result

The concentration of amylase in the given serum sample is ___________ U/L.

Clinical Significance

Reference range: 15–80U/L

Interference: Hemolysis, lipemia

Other methods: 4-NP-G7 method

CHAPTER

18

Estimation of Serum Lipase

Aim: To estimate the concentration of lipase in the given serum sample.

Method: Enzymatic color method.

Principle

$$\text{Colorimetric substrate} \xrightarrow{\text{Lipase}} \underset{\text{(bluish purple color)}}{\text{Glutaric acid + methyl resorufin}}$$

The rate of color formation at 580 nm is proportional to the activity of lipase in the sample.

Procedure

Sample volume: 4 µl
Volume of R1: 160 µl
Volume of R2: 40 µl
Primary wavelength: 580 nm
Secondary wavelength: 660 nm
Assay type: Kinetic assay
Curve type Linear increasing slope
Linearity: 8 to 300 U/L

Calculation

$$\text{Concentration of lipase} = \frac{\text{OD of test} - \text{OD of blank}}{\text{OD of standard} - \text{OD of blank}} \times \text{Conc. of standard}$$

Result

The concentration of lipase in the given serum sample is ____________ U/L.

Clinical Significance

Reference range: 5–60 U/L
Interference: Hemolysis, lipemia
Other methods: Titrimetric method
Turbidimetric method

CHAPTER

19

Estimation of Glucose by Standardisation

Aim: To standardize the stock solution of glucose and to estimate the amount of glucose in the given sample.

Method: Glucose oxidase-peroxidase method (GOD–POD method).

Principle

Glucose present in plasma is oxidized to gluconic acid and hydrogen peroxide by glucose oxidase. Hydrogen peroxide is then converted to water and oxygen by peroxidase. 4 Amino antipyrine accepts oxygen with phenol to give a pink chromogen which is measured at 540 nm.

$$\text{Glu cos e} + O_2 + H_2O \rightarrow \text{Gluconic acid} + H_2O_2$$

$$H_2O_2 \xrightarrow{\text{Peroxidase}} H_2O + [O]$$

$$[O] + 4\ \text{aminoantipyrine} + \text{phenol} \rightarrow \text{Quinoneimine chromogen (pink)}$$

Reagent

Glucose oxidase peroxidase reagent.

Preparation of Stock Solution

1 g %

1 g in 100 ml

1 g of glucose is dissolved in 100 ml of distilled water.

Working Standard or Standard Solution

Standard	*Concentration*	*Stock solution*	*Distilled water*
S1	50 mg/dL	0.5 ml	9.5 ml
S2	100 mg/dL	1 ml	9 ml
S3	150 mg/dL	1.5 ml	8.5 ml
S4	200 mg/dL	2.0 ml	8 ml
S5	250 mg/dL	2.5 ml	7.5 ml

Reagent	*S1*	*S2*	*S3*	*S4*	*S5*	*Blank*	*Std*	*Test*
GOD POD reagent	1000 µl	1000 µl	1000 µl	1000 µl	1000 µl	1000 µl	1000 µl	1000 µl
Distilled water						10 µl		
Std							10 µl	
Test								10 µl
S1	10 µl							
S2		10 µl						
S3			10 µl					
S4				10 µl				
S5					10 µl			

Mix and incubate at 25° for 15 minutes. Take reading at 540 nm (green filter).

S. No	*Samples/standards*	*Optical density*	*Standard OD—blank OD*	*Resulting OD*
1	Blank	B.OD	–	
2	S1 (50 mg/dL)	S1OD	(S1OD–B.OD)	
3	S2 (100 mg/dL)	S2OD	(S2 OD–B.OD)	
4	S3 (150 mg/dL)	S3OD	(S3 OD–B.OD)	
5	S4 (200 mg/dL)	S4OD	(S4 OD–B.OD)	
6	S5 (250 mg/dL)	S5OD	(S5 OD–B.OD)	

Conc of standard = 100 mg/dL
OD of blank =
OD of standard =
OD of test =

Calculation

$$\text{Amount of glucose in test sample} = \frac{\text{OD of test} - \text{OD of blank}}{\text{OD of std} - \text{OD of blank}} \times \text{Conc. of standard}$$

$$= \frac{T - B}{S - B} \times 100$$

Result

The given stock solution of glucose is standardised and the graph is plotted. The concentration of glucose in the given sample is __________ mg/dl.

Reference Values

Fasting blood glucose 70 to 100 mg/dL
Post prandial blood glucose <140 mg/dL
Random blood glucose <140 mg/dL

Clinical Interpretation

Causes of Hyperglycemia

1. Diabetes mellitus
2. Hyperthyroidism

3. Cushing's syndrome
4. Infections

Causes of Hypoglycemia

1. Starvation
2. Hyperinsulinism
3. Hypothyroidism
4. Hypoadrenalism

Other Methods of Glucose Estimation

Enzymatic method

1. Hexokinase method
2. Glucokinase method

Non-enzymatic method

1. Nelson-Somogyi method
2. Asatoor and King method
3. Folin-Wu method
4. O-toluidine method

Note:

1. Preservative—sodium fluoride and potassium oxalate (grey tube)
2. Plasma/serum glucose >> whole blood glucose
3. Arterial glucose 20 to 30 mg/dL >> venous glucose
4. Capillary glucose (glucometer) 20 to 35 mg/dL >> venous glucose

CHAPTER

20

Estimation of Urea by Standardisation

Aim: To standardize the given stock solution of urea and to estimate the amount of urea in the given sample.

Method: DAM–TSC (diacetyl monoxime thiosemicarbazide) method.

Principle

Urea present in the sample reacts with diacetyl monoxime in the hot acidic medium in the presence of ferric chloride to give a pink-colored complex. Thiosemicarbazide acts as a catalyst. The color intensity is directly proportional to the concentration of urea in the sample.

Reagents

- Diacetyl monoxime/thiosemicarbazide reagent (DAM TSC reagent)
- Acid reagent (Mixture of orthophosphoric acid, sulphuric acid and ferric chloride)
- Urea standard 50 mg/dL

Preparation of Stock Solution I

1 gm of urea is dissolved in 100 ml distilled water.

Preparation of Stock Solution II

250 mg in 100 ml (take 25 ml of stock solution I and make up to 75 ml with distilled water).

Working Standards

Standard	*Stock II*	*Distilled water*	*Concentration*
S1	1 ml	9 ml	25 mg/dL
S2	2 ml	8 ml	50 mg/dL
S3	3 ml	7 ml	75 mg/dL
S4	4 ml	6 ml	100 mg/dL
S5	5 ml	5 ml	125 mg/dL

Reagent	*S1*	*S2*	*S3*	*S4*	*S5*	*Blank*	*Std*	*Test*
DAM TSC reagent	1.5 ml	1.5 ml	1.5 ml	1.5 ml	1.5 ml	1.5 ml	1.5 ml	1.5 ml
Acid mixture	1.5 ml	1.5 ml	1.5 ml	1.5 ml	1.5 ml	1.5 ml	1.5 ml	1.5 ml
Distilled water						20 µl		
Std							20 µl	
Test								20 µl
S1	20 µl							
S2		20 µl						
S3			20 µl					
S4				20 µl				
S5					20 µl			

Mix well and place the test tubes in a boiling water bath for 20 minutes. Allow to cool down and take reading at 540 nm (green filter).

S. No	*Samples/standards*	*Optical density*	*Standard OD—blank OD*	*Resulting OD*
1	Blank	B.OD	–	
2	S1 (25 mg/dL)	S1OD	(S1OD–B.OD)	
3	S2 (50 mg/dL)	S2OD	(S2OD–B.OD)	
4	S3 (75 mg/dL)	S3OD	(S3OD–B.OD)	
5	S4 (100 mg/dL)	S4OD	(S4OD–B.OD)	
6	S5 (125 mg/dL)	S5OD	(S5OD–B.OD)	

Conc of standard = 50 mg/dL
OD of blank =
OD of standard =
OD of test =

Calculation

$$\text{Amount of urea in test sample} = \frac{\text{OD of test} - \text{OD of blank}}{\text{OD of std} - \text{OD of blank}} \times \text{Conc. of standard}$$

$$= \frac{T - B}{S - B} \times 100$$

Result

The given stock solution of urea is standardised and the graph is plotted. The concentration of urea in the given sample is __________.

Reference Range

Normal serum urea = 15 to 35 mg/dL

Clinical Interpretation

Increase in serum urea + symptoms = uremia

Causes of Increased Serum Urea

Prerenal Cause

1. Dehydration
2. Shock

Renal Cause

1. Renal failure
2. Acute glomerulonephritis

Postrenal Cause

1. Bladder cancer
2. Urinary tract stones

Other Methods of Urea Estimation

1. Enzymatic method
2. Urease GLDH method.

CHAPTER

21

Estimation of Creatinine by Standardisation

Aim: To standardize the given stock solution of creatinine and to estimate the amount of creatinine in the given sample.

Method: Jaffe's alkaline picrate method.

Principle

Creatinine in the sample reacts with picric acid in an alkaline medium to form red orange-colored compound creatinine picrate. The color intensity is directly proportional to the creatinine concentration in the sample which is measured at 490 nm using a blue filter.

Reagents

0.75 N NaOH

Saturated picric acid

Preparation of Stock Solution I

100 mg of creatinine is dissolved in 100 ml of N/10 HCl.

Preparation of Stock Solution II (10 mg%)

10 ml of stock I + 90 ml of distilled water.

Working Standards

Standard	*Stock II*	*Distilled water*	*Concentration*
S1	1 ml	9 ml	1 mg/dL
S2	2 ml	8 ml	2 mg/dL
S3	3 ml	7 ml	3 mg/dL
S4	4 ml	6 ml	4 mg/dL
S5	5 ml	5 ml	5 mg/dL

Reagent	*S1*	*S2*	*S3*	*S4*	*S5*	*Blank*	*Std*	*Test*
Saturated picric acid	1 ml	1 ml	1 ml	1 ml	1 ml	1 ml	1 ml	1 ml
0.75 N NaOH	1 ml	1 ml	1 ml	1 ml	1 ml	1 ml	1 ml	1 ml
Distilled water						200 µl		
Std							200 µl	
Test								200 µl
S1	200 µl							
S2		200 µl						
S3			200 µl					
S4				200 µl				
S5					200 µl			

Mix well. Incubate at room temperature for 10 minutes. Take reading at 490 nm.

S. No	*Samples/standards*	*Optical density*	*Standard OD—Blank OD*	*Resulting OD*
1	Blank	B.OD	–	
2	S1 (1 mg/dL)	S1OD	(S1OD–B.O.D)	
3	S2 (2 mg/dL)	S2OD	(S2OD–B.OD)	
4	S3 (3 mg/dL)	S3OD	(S3OD–B.OD)	
5	S4 (4 mg/dL)	S4OD	(S4OD–B.OD)	
6	S5 (5 mg/dL)	S5OD	(S5OD–B.OD)	

Conc of standard = 2 mg/dL
OD of blank =
OD of standard =
OD of test =

Calculation

$$\text{Amount of creatinine in test sample} = \frac{\text{OD of test} - \text{OD of blank}}{\text{OD of std} - \text{OD of blank}} \times \text{Conc. of standard}$$

$$= \frac{T - B}{S - B} \times 2$$

Result

The given stock solution of creatinine is standardized and the graph is plotted. The concentration of creatinine in the given sample is ___________.

Reference Range

Normal serum creatinine level in males = 0.7 to 1.4 mg/dL
females = 0.6 to 1.2 mg/dL

Clinical Interpretation

Causes of Increased Serum Creatinine

Prerenal cause:

1. Dehydration
2. Shock

Renal cause

1. Renal failure
2. Acute glomerulonephritis

Postrenal cause:

1. Bladder cancer
2. Urinary tract stones

Other methods of creatinine estimation:

1. Enzymatic method
2. Creatinase method

CHAPTER

22

Test for Carbohydrates

Practicals

Reactions of glucose			
S. No	*Procedure*	*Observation*	*Inference*
1	**Molisch's test** Take 2 ml of sample and add 3 drops of Molisch's reagent. Mix and add 2 ml of concentrated H_2SO_4 along the sides of the tube	A purple ring is obtained at the junction of two liquids	Presence of carbohydrates
2	**Iodine test** Take 2 ml of sample. Add 5 drops of glacial acetic acid and 3 drops of N/50 iodine	No blue color	Absence of polysaccharides
3	**Benedict's test** Take 5 ml of Benedict's reagent. Add 8 drops of sample. Mix and boil for 2 minutes and cool	Red precipitate is formed	Presence of reducing sugar
4	**Barfoed's test** Take 2 ml of Barfoed's reagent. Add 1 ml of sample. Mix and boil for 30 seconds and cool.	Red precipitate is formed	Presence of monosaccharide
5	**Seliwanoff test** Take 2 ml of Seliwanoff reagent and add 3 drops of sample. Boil for 30 seconds	No cherry red color is formed	Absence of ketose
6	**Foulger's test** Take 3 ml of Foulger's reagent. Add 5 drops of sample. Boil for 1 minute and cool	No blue color is formed	Absence of ketose
7	**Osazone test** Take 5 ml of sample in a test tube and add ½ spatula of phenylhydrazine hydrochloride and 1 spatula of sodium acetate and 0.5 ml of glacial acetic acid. Mix well, filter and keep it in a boiling water bath. Transfer crystals to slide and view under the microscope	Needle-shaped yellow crystals of glucosazone is formed	Presence of glucose

Result: Glucose is a reducing monosaccharide, an aldose and forms glucosazone.

CHAPTER

23

Test for Proteins

Experiment	*Observation*	*Inference*
Biuret test: Take 2 ml of protein solution. Add 2 ml of 5% NaOH. Add 2–3 drops of copper sulfate	Purple color is formed	Presence of proteins with 2 or more peptide bonds
Ninhydrin test: To 2 ml of protein solution, add 2–3 drops of ninhydrin and boil	Purple color is formed	Presence of alpha amino acids
Aldehyde test: To 3 ml of protein solution, add 2 drops of 1/500 formalin and 1 drop of 10% mercuric sufate in 10% sulfuric acid. Mix well. Add 3 ml of conc. sulfuric acid along the sides of the test tube held in a slanting position	Purple color ring is formed	Presence of tryptophan
Sulfur test: To 2 ml of protein solution add 2 ml of 40% sodium hydroxide and boil. Then add 5 drops of lead acetate	A black precipitate is formed	Presence of sulfur containing amino acids (cysteine and cystine)

CHAPTER

24

Test for Lipids

SOLUBILITY TEST

Lipids are soluble in non-polar solvents (e.g. chloroform, ether, benzene) and they form one phase. Lipids are insoluble in polar solvents (e.g. water) and they form two phase.

Procedure

Take five test tubes marking A, B, C, D, E. Put 5 ml—water, absolute alcohol, ether, chloroform and benzene one in each test tube. Add 3 to 4 drops of sample in each test tube, shake thoroughly, allow to stand.

Observation

1. In test tube A drops of oils are seen floating on the surface of water
2. In test tube B oil drops settle at the bottom of alcohol
3. In test tubes C, D and E the sample is mixed.

Inference

The sample contains fat, as it is not soluble in water (test tube A) but soluble only in organic solvents (test tube C, D, E) and sinks to the bottom in alcohol (B).

EMULSIFICATION TEST FOR LIPID

Principle

Oil or liquid fat becomes finely divided and is dispersed as minute droplets suspended in the liquid (permanent emulsification) when shaken with oleic acid to form emulsification.

Procedure

Take 3 ml sample in a test tube, add 2 drops of oleic acid, shake well. Add 2 drops of the mixture to another test tube containing 3 ml 10% caustic soda.

Observation

Emulsion is formed

Inference

The test sample contains fat.

SAPONIFICATION TEST

Principle

Saponification is the process of hydrolysis of esters of oils and fats with alkali to form glycerol and salts of fatty acids that is soap.

Procedure

Sample solution (1 ml) + alcoholic NaOH (3 ml) then warm well and stir. Take a piece of the product in water (2 ml) and mix well.

Observation

Froth appears due to soap formation.

Inference

The sample contains fat.

CHAPTER

25

OSPE Stations

QUALITATIVE TESTS

Heat coagulation test

1. Identify the test. (1 mark)
   Heat coagulation test for proteins
2. Write the principle of the test. (3 marks)
   On heating, proteins lose their shell of hydration and get coagulated. The coagulum gets intensified by adding acetic acid.

Benedict's test

1. Identify the test. (1 mark)
   Benedict's test for reducing sugars
2. Write the principle of the test. (3 marks)
   Under alkaline conditions sugars form enediols which reduces cupric hydroxide to cuprous hydroxide which on heating is further converted to cuprous oxide which may be green, yellow, orange or brick red precipitate depending on the amount of reducing sugars present in it.

Heat coagulation test

1. Identify the test. (1 mark)
2. What does the test detect? (1 mark)—protein
3. Write the procedure of the test. (3 marks)—fill 3/4th of the test tube with a protein solution and heat the upper 1/3rd of the solution.

Rothera's test

1. Identify the test. (1 mark)
2. What does the test detect? (1 mark)—ketone bodies
3. Write the principle of the test. (3 marks) acetone and acetoacetic acid reacts with an alkaline solution of sodium nitroprusside to form a purple colored complex.

Jaffe's test

1. Identify the test. (1 mark)
2. What does the test detect? (1 mark)—creatinine
3. Write the principle of the test. (3 marks)—creatinine reacts with alkaline picrate to form creatinine picrate which is an orange-red complex.

Hay's test

1. Identify the test. (1 mark)
2. What does the test detect? (1 mark)—bile salts
3. Write the principle of the test. (3 marks)—bile salts reduce the surface tension

Nutrition

Indian gooseberry/lemon

1. What is the vitamin-rich in this food? (1 mark)—vitamin C
2. Mention any two functions of that vitamin (2 marks)—collagen formation, wound healing, iron absorption
3. Mention any two deficiency manifestations of this vitamin. (2 marks)—scurvy, bleeding gums

Milk

1. What is the mineral rich in this food? (1 mark)—calcium
2. What is the reference range of that mineral in serum? (1 mark)—9–11 mg/dl
3. Mention any three functions of that mineral. (3 marks)—bone and teeth, blood coagulation, muscle contraction

Jaggery

1. What is the mineral-rich in this food? (1 mark)—iron
2. Name any two functions of the mineral. (2 marks)—haemoglobin, myoglobin, iron-containing enzymes
3. Mention any two deficiency manifestations of the mineral. (2 marks)—anemia, lethargy, growth retardation, breathlessness, cardiac failure

Carrot

1. What is the vitamin-rich in this food? (1 mark)
   Vitamin A
2. Write any two functions and deficiency manifestations of this vitamin. (3 marks)
   Vision, cell differentiation. Night blindness, corneal xerosis, Bitot's spots, corneal ulcers

Instruments

Centrifuge

1. Identify the instrument. (1 mark)
2. List two of its uses. (2 marks)—serum separation, subcellular fractionation
3. Write its principle of working. (2 marks)—separation and sedimentation due to relative centrifugal force expressed as sedimentation coefficient

pH Meter

1. Identify the instrument. (1 mark)
2. What is it used for? (1 mark)—measuring the pH of buffers and solutions
3. Write its principle of working. (3 marks)—when a glass membrane separates two different solutions having different pH, a potential difference is found to be present between the surfaces of the glass. The potential is measured against a standard calomel electrode.

Colorimeter

1. Identify the instrument. (1 mark)
2. What is the wavelength range of the visible light spectrum? (1 mark)—300–700 nm
3. Write its principle of working. (3 marks)—Beer's Law—when a beam of monochromatic light passes through the solution, the absorbance is directly proportional to the concentration of the substance in the solution. Lambert's law—Absorbance is directly proportional to path length.

Flame Photometry

1. Identify the instrument. (1 mark)
2. What is it used for? (1 mark)—measure serum electrolytes sodium, potassium
3. Write its principle of working. (3 marks)—diluted serum is sprayed by means of an atomiser into a Bunsen flame. Colored vapours are produced for different elements like Na and K due to emission spectrum. Emitted rays fall on phototube and produce a current which deflects the galvanometer.

ELECTROPHORESIS

1. Identify the band 'X'. (2 marks) —Albumin band
2. Name the bands present in serum protein electrophoresis. (3 marks)—Albumin, α_1, α_2, β_1, β_2, γ bands
3. What is the principle of electrophoresis? (5 marks)—separation of proteins by migration of charged ions under electric field and their mass.

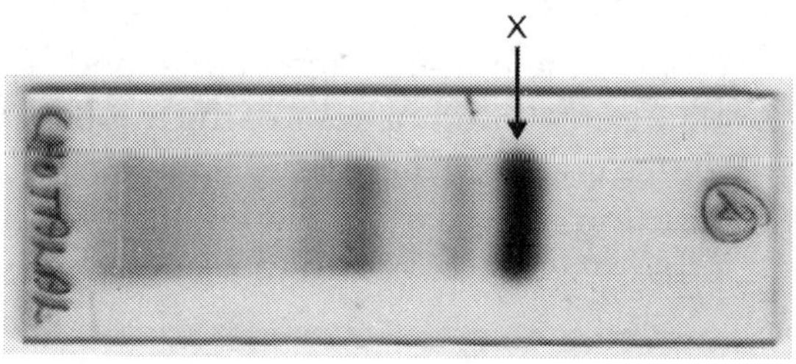

Semi-automated Analyser

1. Identify the instrument (1 mark)
2. What is it used for? (1 mark)
   Used for quantitative estimation of glucose, urea, creatinine, cholesterol, bilirubin, total protein, albumin
3. Tabulate the difference between semiautomated and fully automated analyser (3 marks)

Semi-autoanalyser	*Fully automated analyser*
1. Manual pipetting of sample and reagents	1. Automated pipetting of sample and reagents
2. Less accuracy and precision	2. High accuracy and precision
3. Long turn around time, delayed reports	3. Short turn around time, quick results
4. Less expensive	4. Highly expensive
5. Less maintenance	5. Requires more maintenance

BMI

An individual weighs 80 kg and is 160 cm tall. Write the formula and calculate his BMI. (4 marks)

BMI = Weight in kg/height in m^2

80/1.6 × 1.6 = 31.2 kg/m^2

BMI Case

An individual weighs 80 kg and is 160 cm tall:

a. Calculate his BMI and write the formula. (3 marks)
b. Interpret his BMI. (1 mark)
c. Write the classification of BMI. (3 marks)
d. List the factors affecting BMI (1 mark)
e. Name any FOUR anthropometric indices.

  a. BMI = Weight in kg/height in m^2
  $80/1.6 \times 1.6 = 31.2$ kg/m^2
  b. Obese
  c. Underweight: <18.5 kg/m^2
  Normal: 18.5–24.9 kg/m^2
  Overweight: 25.0–29.9 kg/m^2
  Obese: $\geq$30.0 kg/m^2
  Extreme obesity: $\geq$40.0 kg/m^2
  d. Age, sex, temperature, exercise, fever, thyroid hormones
  e. Weight, mid arm circumference (MAC), BMI (body mass index), waist circumference (WC), waist hip ratio (WHR)

Vitamin A

a. Identify the nutritional deficiency in the given picture and the deficient nutrient. (2 marks)
b. List any four clinical signs of malnutrition. (4 marks)
c. List any four biochemical tests of malnutrition (4 marks)

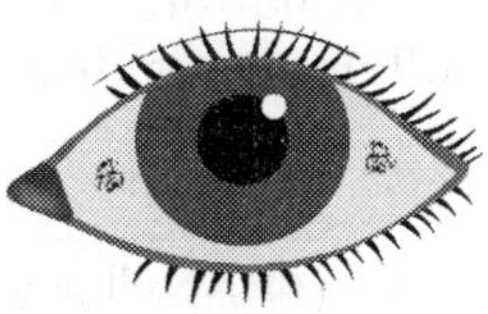

Key

a. Bitot's spot, vitamin A deficiency
b. Dry brittle hair, thyroid enlargement, glossitis, dental caries, dry scaly skin, spoon shaped nails, knock knee, bow legs, muscle wasting
c. Serum protein, serum albumin, serum transferrin, serum vitamin D levels, serum vitamin B_{12} levels, serum iron, serum ferritin, serum calcium.

CLINICAL CASES

CARDIAC CASE 1

A 48-year-old man came to the casualty with complaints of chest pain and vomiting for the past 4 hours. He gave history of consuming alcohol the previous evening. He was anxious saying that his father died of myocardial infarction at the age of 65. On examination, he was anxious. Pulse-86/min; BP-140/90 mm Hg. ECG was normal. Blood was drawn for biochemical analysis.

1. Name any FIVE cardiac biomarkers that can be estimated in this patient. (5 marks)—CK-MB, troponin T, troponin I, AST, LDH, myoglobin
2. Mention any FIVE risk factors for cardiovascular diseases. (5 marks)—age, male, smoking, obesity, high BP, high cholesterol, low HDL

CARDIAC CASE 2

On examination, he was profusely sweating. His blood pressure was 160/100 mmHg. ECG showed S–T segment elevation. He was suspected to have myocardial infarction. A blood sample taken for biochemical analysis showed:

Serum CK	1160 U/L (10–80 U/L)
Serum CK-MB	270 U/L (5–25 U/L)
Serum AST	380 U/L (8–20 U/L)
Serum LDH	350 U/L (100–200 U/L)

1. What is the other cardiac biomarker that can be estimated in this patient? (2 marks)
   troponin T, troponin I
2. Mention any three risk factors for myocardial infarction. (3 marks)
   Elderly age, obesity, atherosclerosis, hypertension, smoking, high cholesterol, low HDL.

LFT CASE 1

A 24-year-old male was admitted with fever, nausea and abdominal pain. On examination, he was slightly jaundiced. The biochemical tests done showed the following results.

Serum bilirubin (total)	3.8 mg/dL
Serum direct bilirubin (conjugated)	2.1 mg/dL
Serum indirect bilirubin (unconjugated)	1.7 mg/dL
Aspartate amino transferase	282 IU/L
Alanine amino transferase	390 IU/L
Serum alkaline phosphatase	178 IU/L
Urinary findings: Bile pigments Bile salts	 +++ +

1. Give your interpretation of the bilirubin levels in this patient. (3 marks)
   Total bilirubin is elevated
   Direct bilirubin is elevated
   Indirect bilirubin is elevated
2. What is the test used to detect bile salts in urine? Write its principle. (2 marks)
   Hay's test

Bile salts act as surfactants and reduce the surface tension and hence the sulfur powder sinks to the bottom of the tube.

Bile salts are sodium taurocholate and sodium taurochenodeoxycholate.

LFT CASE 2

A person was referred to the surgical OP with a three months history of epigastric pain, radiating to the back and weight loss. He gave history of passing dark colored urine and pale stools.

Lab investigations showed:	
Serum bilirubin (total)	25.0 mg/dL
Serum direct bilirubin (conjugated)	20.0 mg/dL
Serum Indirect bilirubin (unconjugated)	5.0 mg/dL
Urinary findings:	
Bile pigments	+++
Bile salts	++
Urobilinogen	Absent
Feces	Clay colored stools

1. What are the liver enzyme markers that can be estimated in this patient? (3 marks)
   AST, ALT, ALP, GGT
2. What is the test used to detect bile pigments in urine? (2 marks)
   Fouchet's test
3. Write the principle of the test for bile pigments. (5 marks)

The precipitate of barium sulfate absorbs the bile pigments. Ferric chloride present in Fouchet's reagent oxidises bilirubin to biliverdin

RFT CASE 1

A 56-year-old man was admitted with loss of appetite, nausea, vomiting, difficulty in breathing and fatigue. History revealed that he was diagnosed 5 years back with hypertension and kidney failure. On examination, his pulse rate was 64/min, BP was 170/100 mm Hg. No other abnormality was detected.

Laboratory investigations showed:	
Random blood glucose	140 mg/dL
Blood urea	65 mg/dL
Serum creatinine	2.4 mg/dL
Serum sodium	139 mEq/L
Serum potassium	4.9 mEq/L
Urine sugar	Nil
Urine albumin	3+

1. What are the abnormal results in the given laboratory report? (3 marks)
   Urea is elevated
   Creatinine is elevated
   Proteinuria present
2. Name the test used to detect albumin in urine. (2 marks)
   Sulfosalicylic acid test, heat coagulation test, dipstick test

RFT CASE 2

A 50-year-old hypertensive man came with history of sore throat and fever. On examination he was afebrile, BP 140/94 mmHg, pulse 80/min. Facial and lower limb edema was present. He was diagnosed to have nephrotic syndrome. Investigation results are as:

Fasting blood glucose	280 mg/dL
Blood urea	120 mg/dL
Serum creatinine	2.0 mg/dL
Serum albumin	2 g/dL
Serum cholesterol	280 mg/dL
Urine sugar	4+
Urine albumin	3+

1. What is the method of creatinine estimation in serum? (1 mark)

   Modified Jaffe's method
2. What is the test used to detect urine sugar? (1 mark)

   Benedict's test
3. Write the principle for the test used to detect urine sugar. (3 marks)

   Under alkaline conditions sugars form enediols which reduce cupric hydroxide to cuprous hydroxide which on heating is further converted to cuprous oxide which may be green, yellow or red precipitate that indicates the presence of reducing sugars.

RFT CASE 3

A 50-year-old hypertensive man came with history of sore throat and fever. On examination he was afebrile, BP 140/94 mmHg, pulse 80/min. Facial and lower limb edema was present. He was diagnosed to have nephrotic syndrome. Investigation results are as:

Fasting blood glucose	280 mg/dL
Blood urea	120 mg/dL
Serum creatinine	2.0 mg/dL
Serum albumin	2 g/dL
Serum cholesterol	280 mg/dL
Urine sugar	4+
Urine albumin	3+

1. What is the method of creatinine estimation in serum? (2 marks)—Modified Jaffe's method
2. What is the test used to detect urine sugar? (2 marks)—Benedicts test
3. What is the reference range of creatinine in serum? (1 mark)—0.6–1.2 mg/dL

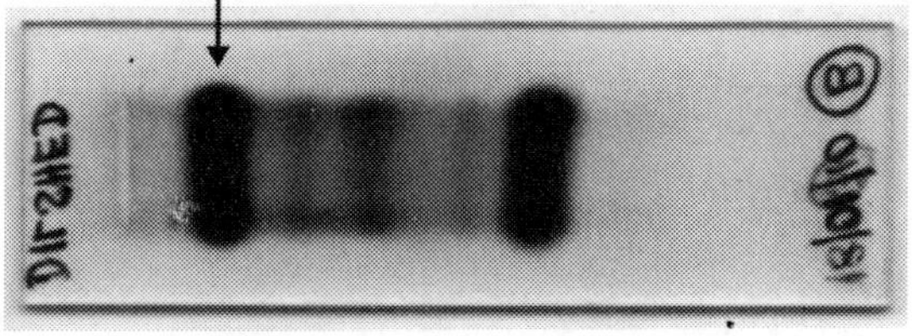

Serum electrophoresis pattern

MULTIPLE MYELOMA CASE

1. Identify the band 'X'. (2 marks)
   M band in multiple myeloma
2. What is the principle of protein electrophoresis? (3 marks)
   Proteins and amino acids carry a negative charge in an alkaline medium. When subjected to the electric field, proteins get separated based on their charge and molecular weight. The movement of the ions is dependent on the current strength, pH of the buffer and temperature.

Spotters for MLT

Centrifuge

1. Identify the instrument
   Centrifuge
2. List two of its uses
   a. Separation of serum, plasma
   b. Separation of protein free filtrate
   c. Fractionation of subcellular organelles

Molisch test

1. Name the test.
2. What does the test detects?
   Presence of carbohydrates

Benedict's test

1. Name the test.
2. What is the composition of the reagent?
   Sodium carbonate, sodium citrate, copper sulfate

Egg

1. What is the major nutrient present in this food?
   Proteins
2. Name any two essential amino acids.
   Methionine, phenylalanine, tryptophan, threonine, isoleucine, leucine, lysine

Urinometer

1. Identify the instrument.
2. What is the normal specific gravity of urine?
   1.003–1.030

Colorimeter

1. Identify the instrument.
2. What is the wavelength range of the visible light spectrum?
   300–700 nm

Sulphur powder

1. Name the chemical.
2. Name the test in which it is used.
   Hay's test

OGTT chart

1. What is the graph displayed?
2. Write the reference range for fasting and postprandial blood glucose levels.
   Fasting: 70–100 mg/dl
   Postprandial: 120–140 mg/dl

Carrot

1. What is the vitamin-rich in this food?
   Vitamin A
2. Write any two functions of this vitamin.
   Vision, Cell Differentiation

Serum tube

1. Name the different types of anticoagulant tubes.
   EDTA tube, sodium citrate tube, heparin tube, fluoride tube
2. What is the anticoagulant of choice for glucose estimation?
   Grey tube (contains sodium fluoride and potassium oxalate)

Milk

1. What is the mineral rich in this food?
   Calcium.
2. What is the reference range of that mineral in serum?
   9–11 mg/dL

Rothera's test

1. Name the test.
2. What does the test detect?
   Presence of ketone bodies (acetone, acetoacetate)

Flame photometry

1. Identify the instrument
2. What is it used for?
   Estimation of serum electrolytes

pH meter

1. Identify the instrument.
2. What is it used for?
   Measurement of pH of urine and buffer solutions

Heat coagulation test

1. Name the test.
2. What does the test detect?
   Presence of proteins

Jaffe's test

1. Name the test.
2. What does the test detect?
   Presence of creatinine

Seliwanoff's test

1. Name the test.
2. What does the test detect?
   Presence of ketoses

Hay's test

1. Name the test.
2. What does the test detect?
   Presence of bile salts

Electrophoresis apparatus

1. Identify the instrument.
2. What is it used for?
   Separation of serum proteins, urine proteins, lipoproteins, hemoglobin separation

Indian gooseberry

1. What is the vitamin-rich in this food?
   Vitamin C
2. Mention one function of that vitamin.
   Collagen formation, antioxidant

Cobas immunoassay analyser

1. What is the principle of working of this analyser?
   Electrochemiluminescent immunoassay (ECLIA)
2. Name any four investigations done in this analyser.
   A. Thyroid function tests—FT_4, TSH
   B. Tumour markers—beta HCG, CA-125, total PSA
   C. Inflammatory markers—IL-6, ferritin, procalcitonin
   D. Cardiac markers—troponin-T

Fully automated chemistry analyser

1. What are the types of fully automated analysers?
   Batch analyser and random access analyser
2. Give any two advantages of this over the semiautoanalyser.
   A. Can process a large number of samples
   B. Accurate and precise results

C. Short turn around time

D. Can store quality control data and patient data

ABG analyser

1. What is the principle of working of this analyser?
   Ion selective electrode method
2. What are the parameters included in ABG analysis?
   pH, pO_2, pCO_2, HCO_3 (bicarbonate), electrolytes

Electrolyte analyser

1. What is the principle of working of this analyser?
   Ion selective electrode method
2. Give two uses of this analyser.
   Electrolyte estimation, therapeutic drug monitoring (TDM).

CHAPTER

26

Viva Voce Questions and Answers

Q1. What are enzymes?

Ans: Enzymes are biocatalysts.

Q2. Give examples of coenzymes.

Ans: NAD, NADP, metal ions like calcium, magnesium, folic acid.

Q3. What is glycolysis?

Ans: It is the breakdown of glucose for energy.

Q4. What is the storage form of glucose?

Ans: Glycogen

Q5. Where is glycogen stored?

Ans: Liver, muscle

Q6. What is the use of the HMP pathway?

Ans: Ribose synthesis for DNA and RNA, NADPH synthesis for lipid metabolism.

Q7. Name the hormones regulating blood glucose level

Ans: Hypoglycemic—insulin, hyperglycemic—glucagon, growth hormone, adrenaline.

Q8. What is fasting blood glucose?

Ans: Blood glucose measured after 8–10 hours of fasting.

Q9. What is postprandial blood glucose?

Ans: Blood glucose measured after 2 hours of food intake.

Q10. What is HbA1c?

Ans: It is glycated haemoglobin.

Q11. What are the advantages of HbA1c?

Ans: It denotes the long-term control of blood glucose for the past 3 months, patient need not come in fasting, and more than 6.5% is diagnostic of diabetes mellitus.

Q12. What is diabetes mellitus?

Ans: It is a state of hyperglycemia due to insulin deficiency or insulin resistance.

Q13. What are the criteria to diagnose diabetes mellitus?

Ans: Fasting glucose >125 mg/dL, postprandial glucose >200 mg/dL, HbA1c >6.5%.

Q14. What is urea?

Ans: It is the end product of protein catabolism.

Q15. Where is urea synthesized?

Ans: In the liver by urea cycle.

Q16. How is urea excreted?

Ans: In urine

Q17. Name some amino acids.

Ans: Glycine, serine, threonine, valine, leucine, isoleucine, lysine, cysteine, methionine, phenylalanine, tyrosine, tryptophan, histidine, glutamate, glutamine, aspartate, asparagine, arginine.

Q18. Classify lipids.

Ans: Simple lipids—triglycerides or fats, waxes
Compound lipids—phospholipids
Derived lipids—fatty acids, steroids.

Q19. What are the functions of lipids?

Ans: Storage form of energy
Structural component of cell membrane
Insulation of neurons
Synthesis of steroid hormones
Give shape and contour to the body
Protect internal organs
Helps in the absorption of fat-soluble vitamins.

Q20. What are the functions of vitamin A?

Ans: Dim vision, Wald's visual cycle, cell differentiation.

Q21. What are the functions of vitamin D?

Ans: Bone and teeth mineralization, immunity, prevention of diabetes and hypertension.

Q22. What are the functions of vitamin K?

Ans: Activation of clotting factors 2, 7, 9, 10.

Q23. What is the function of vitamin E?

Ans: Antioxidant

Q24. What is the function of B complex vitamins?

Ans: Act as coenzymes for metabolism, synthesis and maturation of RBCs and heme, growth and differentiation, myelination of nerves and nerve conduction.

Q25. Mention the functions of vitamin C.

Ans: Redox reactions, collagen synthesis, iron absorption, immunity, antioxidant, prevent cancer.

Q26. Deficiency of vitamin C.

Ans: Scurvy, bleeding gums, internal bleeding, soft bones and nails, anemia.

Q27. What are the functions of calcium?

Ans: Activation of enzymes, muscle contraction, nerve conduction, secretion of insulin, second messenger, blood clotting, heart pumping (contraction), calcification of bones and teeth.

Q28. What is the normal blood pH?

Ans: 7.35–7.45 decrease in pH is called acidosis, increase in pH is called alkalosis.

Q29. What is a buffer?

Ans: A buffer is a substance that resists any change in pH.

Q30. What are the types of buffers in the body?

Ans: Blood buffers, respiratory buffers, renal buffers.

Q31. Give examples of blood buffers.

Ans: Bicarbonate buffer, phosphate buffer, haemoglobin buffer, protein buffer.

Q32. Name some pH indicators.

Ans: Phenolphthalein, methyl orange, methyl red.

Q33. What kind of sample is collected for blood gas analysis?

Ans: Arterial sample.

Q34. What are the parameters measured in blood gas analysis?

Ans: pH, pO_2, pCO_2, bicarbonate.

Q35. What are the types of protein energy malnutrition?

Ans: Marasmus, kwashiorkar.

SECTION

IV

Clinical Biochemistry

1. Liver Function Test
2. Renal Function Tests (RFT)
3. Renal Clearance Tests
4. Proteinuria
5. Thyroid Function Tests
6. Gastric Function Tests
7. Pancreatic Function Tests
8. Oral Glucose Tolerance Test (OGTT)
9. Clinical Enzymology Enzymes Used as Cardiac Markers
10. Lipid Profile
11. Cerebrospinal Fluid Analysis
12. Pleural Fluid Analysis
13. Arterial Blood Gas Analysis
14. Plasma Proteins
15. Fibrinogen
16. Prothrombin Time (PT)
17. Applications of Radioisotopes
18. Stone Analysis

CHAPTER

1

Liver Function Test

Functions of Liver

1. Metabolism of carbohydrates, lipids and proteins
2. Storage of glycogen, vitamins
3. Synthesis of albumin, clotting factors
4. Excretion of bile salts, bile pigments
5. Detoxification.

Indications of Liver Function Tests

1. Jaundice
2. Liver diseases
3. Any chronic illness
4. Patients taking treatment for HIV, TB
5. Annual checkup for diabetes mellitus and hypertensive patients.

Classification of liver function tests based on function of liver

Excretory function	Synthetic function	Liver enzymes	Special tests
1. Serum bilirubin 2. Urine bile salts 3. Urine urobilinogen	1. Total protein 2. Albumin 3. Albumin globulin ratio (A:G) 4. Prothrombin time	1. AST—aspartate transaminase 2. ALT—alanine transaminase 3. ALP—alkaline phosphatase 4. GGT—gammaglutamyl transferase	1. Ceruloplasmin 2. Ferritin 3. Alpa fetoprotein (AFP)

Tests for Excretory Functions of the Liver

Bilirubin

Normal level of serum total bilirubin—0.2 to 0.8 mg/dL

Total bilirubin → Direct bilirubin—conjugated
Total bilirubin → Indirect bilirubin—unconjugated bilirubin

Normal level of direct bilirubin: 0 to 0.2 mg/dL

Indirect bilirubin = Total bilirubin—direct bilirubin

Normal level of indirect bilirubin: 0.2–0.6 mg/dL

Method of Serum Bilirubin Estimation

1. Diazo method
2. Jendrassik-grof method

Principle: van den Bergh's reaction

Serum total bilirubin >1 mg/dL—hyperbilirubinemia
>2 mg/dL—jaundice

Tests for Detection of Urine Bilirubin

- Fouchet's test
- Gmelin's test

Test for Detection of Urine Bile Salts (Hay's Test)

1. Bile salts are sodium and potassium salts of conjugated bile acids
2. Primary bile acids are cholic acid and chenodeoxy cholic acid
3. Conjugated bile acids are bile acids conjugated with glycine or taurine, e.g. glycocholic acid.

Test for Detection of Urine Urobilinogen (Ehrlich's Test)

1. Urobilinogen is a normal constituent of urine.
2. Urine urobilinogen is absent in obstructive jaundice.

Test for Dubin-Johnson syndrome: Bromosulphthalcin test (BSP test).

Tests for Synthetic Functions of Liver

1. Serum total protein:
   - Normal level: 6 to 8 g/dL
   - Estimated by Biuret method
2. Serum albumin:
   - Normal level: 3.5 to 5 g/dL
   - Estimated by BCG method
3. Serum globulin = Total protein–Albumin
   - Normal level: 1.5 to 3 g/dL
4. Albumin globulin ratio (A:G) = 1.5:1
5. Serum protein electrophoresis

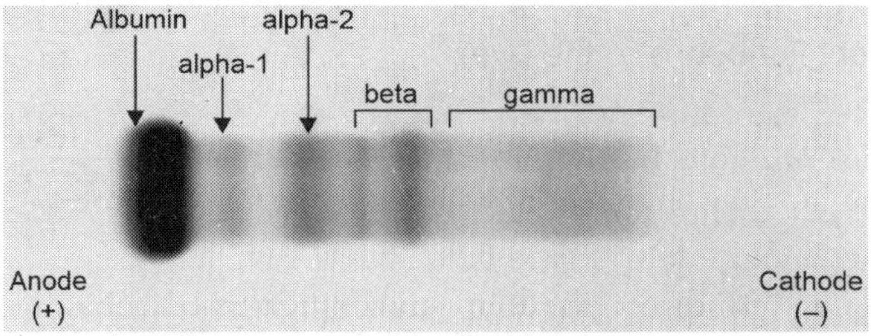

6. **Prothrombin time:** Prothrombin time is the time taken by the blood to clot after adding calcium and tissue thromboplastin.

Normal prothrombin time = 15 to 18 seconds
INR = International normalised ratio
Normal level of INR –1 to 1.2

$$INR = \left(\frac{PT\ (Test)}{PT\ (Control)}\right)^{ISI}$$

ISI—International sensitivity index

Uses of INR

1. To adjust the dose of anticoagulants
2. In patients who underwent cardiac surgery
3. In chronic liver disease

Liver Enzymes

1. Aspartate transaminase (AST) or SGOT:
   Normal level: 10–45 IU/L
   AST is found in the liver, heart, muscle and brain
2. Alanine transaminase (ALT) or SGPT:
   Normal level—5–40 IU/L
   ALT is specific to the liver
   Method of estimation of AST and ALT: IFCC Kinetic method
   AST and ALT are increased in:
   - Hepatitis
   - Liver cirrhosis
   - Alcoholic liver disease
3. Alkaline phosphatase (ALP):
   Normal level—30–150 IU/L
   ALP is present in the bile duct
   ALP is increased in obstructive jaundice
4. Gamma glutamyl transferase (GGT):
   Normal level—10–50 IU/L
   GGT is increased in:
   - Obstructive jaundice
   - Alcoholic liver disease
5. 5′ Nucleotidase (5′ NT) is increased in obstructive jaundice

Special Tests to Assess Liver Function

1. Serum ceruloplasmin
   Normal level: 20–40 mg/dL
   Decreased in Wilson's disease
2. Serum ferritin
   Normal level: 15–400 mg/dL
   Used as an inflammatory marker and in the diagnosis of anaemia
3. Alpha-fetoprotein (AFP)
   Normal level: 0–4 IU/mL
   Increased in malignant neoplasm of liver

Laboratory tests to differentiate the types of jaundice				
S. No	*Tests*	*Hemolytic jaundice*	*Hepatic jaundice*	*Obstructive jaundice*
1	Total bilirubin	Increased	Increased	Increased
2	Indirect bilirubin	Increased	Increased	Normal
3	Direct bilirubin	Normal	Increased	Increased
4	Total protein	Decreased	Decreased	Decreased
5	Albumin	Decreased	Decreased	Decreased
6	AST	Normal	Increased	Mild increase/normal
7	ALT	Normal	Increased	Mild increase/normal
8	ALP	Normal	Mild increase/normal	Increased
9	Urine bile salts	Absent	Absent/present	Present
10	Urine bile pigments	Absent	Absent/present	Present
11	Urine urobilinogen	Increased	Normal/reduced	Absent

Van den Bergh Test

Bilirubin is estimated by van den Bergh test
Diazotised sulfanilic acid = Sulfanilic acid in HCl + sodium nitrite

I. Direct van den Bergh Positive

Bilirubin + diazotised sulfanilic acid → Purple color (direct bilirubin)

II. Indirect van den Bergh Positive

$$\text{Bilirubin + diazotised sulfanilic acid} \xrightarrow[\text{Accelerator}]{\text{Alcohol}} \text{Purple colour (indirect bilirubin)}$$

- Direct bilirubin → Conjugated bilirubin
- Indirect bilirubin → Unconjugated bilirubin
- Total bilirubin = Direct bilirubin + indirect bilirubin

III. Biphasic van den Bergh Reaction

$$\text{Purple colour (direct)} \xrightarrow{\text{Alcohol}} \text{Deep purple colour (indirect)}$$

Interpretation

- Increased direct bilirubin → Obstructive jaundice
- Increased indirect bilirubin → Hemolytic jaundice
- Biphasic reaction → Hepatocellular jaundice

CHAPTER

2

Renal Function Tests (RFT)

Functions of Kidneys

1. Excretion of metabolic waste products like urea
2. Activation of vitamin D
3. Maintains the water balance
4. Maintains electrolyte balance
5. Maintains blood pH and acid–base balance

Indications

1. In cases of proteinuria
2. In cases of diabetes mellitus and hypertension
3. In cases of long-term drug intake

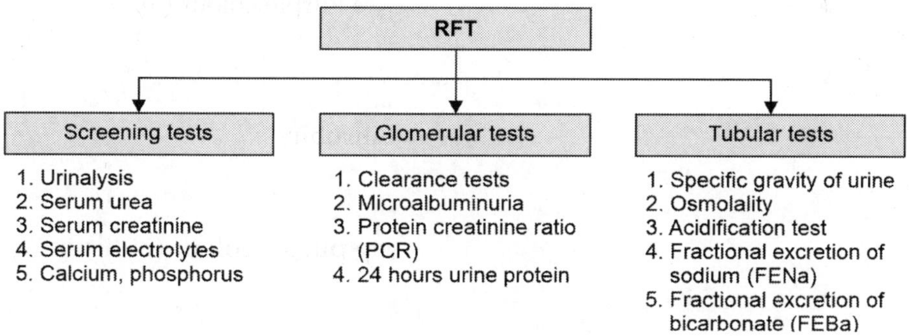

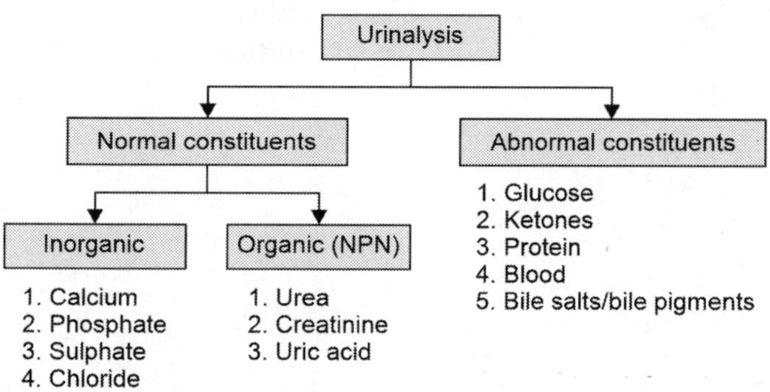

Physical Properties of Urine

1. Colour—amber
2. Volume—1.5 to 2 litres
3. pH—4 to 9
4. Specific gravity—0.003 to 0.030
5. Appearance—clear

S. No	*Parameters*	*Method of estimation*	*Reference range*
1	Serum urea	Urease glutamate dehydrogenase method	15 to 35 mg/dL
2	Serum creatinine	Modified Jaffe's kinetic method	0.6 to 1.2 mg/dL (females) 0.7 to 1.4 mg/dL (males)
3	Serum electrolytes Sodium Potassium Chloride	ISE method	 135 to 145 mEq/L 3.5 to 5 mEq/L 96 to 106 mEq/L
4	Microalbuminuria	Turbidimetry	30 to 300 mg/day
5	Protein creatinine ratio	Microprotein (pyrogallol red method)	<0.2
6	Proteinuria	Dipstick method/pyrogallol red method	<150 mg/day
7	Serum osmolality	Calculation (2 × Na) + Glucose/18 + Urea/6	285–300 mOsm/kg

CHAPTER

3

Renal Clearance Tests

Definition of Clearance

The volume of plasma from which the substance is completely cleared by the kidneys per unit time.

$$\text{Clearance} = \text{GFR (glomerular filtration rate)}$$
$$= \frac{UV}{P}$$

U—concentration of substance in urine (mg/dL)
P—concentration of substance in plasma (mg/dL)
V—volume of urine (ml/min)

Gold standard clearance → Inulin clearance
Silver standard clearance → EDTA - Cr^{51} clearance
Bronze standard clearance → Creatinine clearance
Not useful → Urea clearance

Markers of clearance

Endogenous	Exogenous
1. Creatinine	1. Inulin
2. Cystatin C	2. EDTA – Cr^{15}
3. Urea	3. Iohexol

Creatinine clearance is affected by:

1. Age
2. Sex
3. Muscle mass
4. Exercise
5. Diet

Calculation of Estimated GFR (eGFR)

1. **MDRD equation:**
   - Creatinine
   - Age
   - Sex
   - Race
2. **Cockroft gault formula:**
   - Plasma creatinine
   - Age
   - Weight
   - Sex
3. **CKD—EPI formula:**
   - Plasma creatinine
   - Age
   - Sex
   - Race

CHAPTER

4

Proteinuria

INTRODUCTION TO PROTEINURIA

- It refers to loss of proteins in urine
- Persistent proteinuria is a marker of renal dysfunction

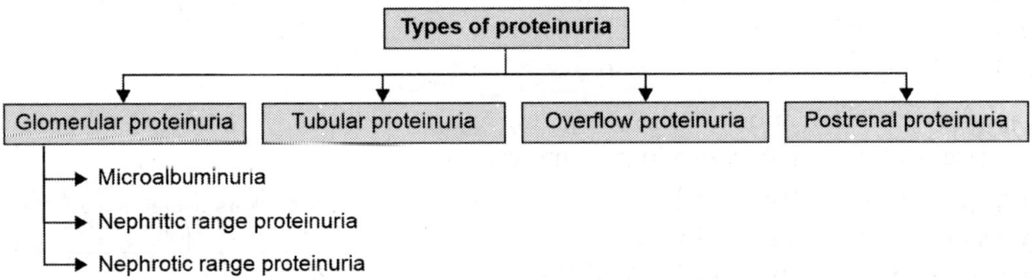

Glomerular Proteinuria

It is due to damage to the glomerulus:

Types	*Range of proteinuria*
Microalbuminuria	30–300 mg/day
Nephritic range	500–1500 mg/day
Nephrotic range	> 3000 mg/day

Overflow Proteinuria

Increased levels of protein in blood overflows in urine

Example: Hemoglobinuria, Bence-Jones proteinuria

Postrenal Proteinuria

It is due to urinary tract infections and urinary tract tumours.

Others

1. Orthostatic proteinuria—due to prolonged standing.
2. Functional proteinuria—fever, pregnancy.

CHAPTER

5

Thyroid Function Tests

Functions of Thyroid Hormones

1. Increase heat production
2. Increase BMR
3. Increase protein breakdown
4. Increase glucose levels
5. Decrease cholesterol levels

Indications for TFT

1. Obesity
2. Infertility
3. Voice change

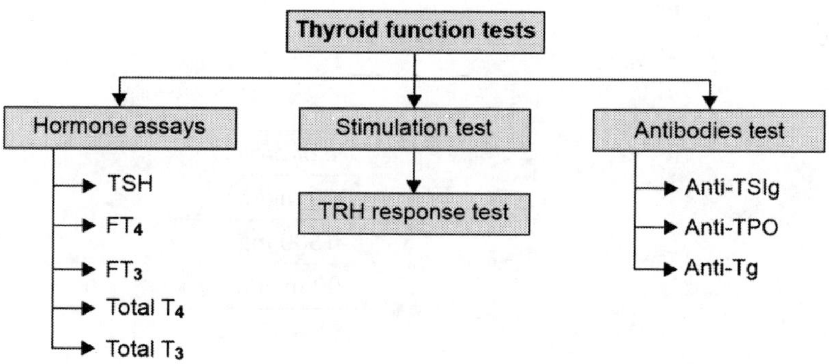

Hormone Assays

- TSH—thyroid stimulating hormone
- FT_4—free thyroxine (0.03%) of total T_4
- FT_3—free T_3 (0.3%) of total T_3
- Free hormone is the functionally active hormone

Method of Assay

1. ECLIA—electrochemiluminescence immunoassay
2. ELISA—enzyme-linked immunoassay

3. RIA—radioimmunoassay
4. ELFA—enzyme linked fluorescent assay

Other Investigations

1. Serum cholesterol
2. RAIU—radioactive iodine uptake
3. Thyroid scan

Laboratory Findings in Thyroid Disorders

S. No	*Disorder*	*FT_4*	*FT_3*	*TSH*
1	Primary hypothyroidism	↓	↓	↑↑
2	Secondary hypothyroidism	↓	↓	↓
3	Primary hyperthyroidism	↑	↑	↓↓
4	Secondary hyperthyroidism	↑	↑	↑
5	Euthyroid	N	N	N

Reference Range

Serum FT_4—0.9–1.7 ng/dL
Serum TSH—0.4–4.2 uIU/mL

CHAPTER

6

Gastric Function Tests

Functions of Stomach

1. HCl secretion
2. Mucous secretion
3. Enzymes secretion

Indications for Gastric Function Test

1. Gastric ulcer
2. Gastrinoma (ZES: Zollinger-Ellison syndrome)

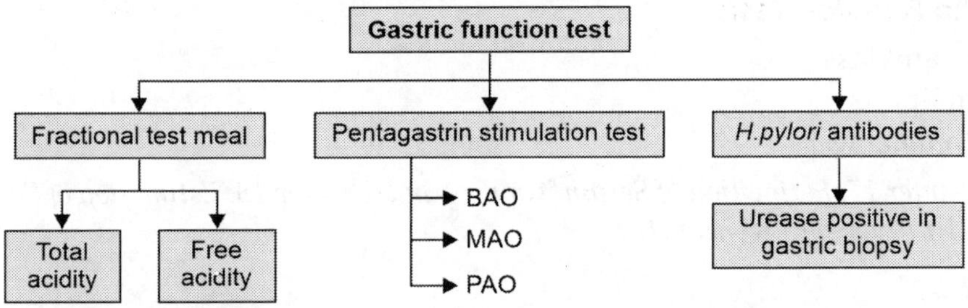

BAO : Basal acid output
MAO : Maximal acid output
PAO : Peak acid output

CHAPTER

7

Pancreatic Function Tests

Pancreatic Juice

- Secretion—1000 to 2500 ml/day
- Contains bicarbonate and enzymes

Indications for Pancreatic Function Tests

1. Acute pancreatitis
2. Chronic pancreatitis
3. Carcinoma of pancreas

Pancreatic Function Tests

1. Serum amylase
2. Serum lipase
3. Lundh meal test

Refer to Chapter 17: Estimation of Serum Amylase and Chapter 18: Estimation of Serum Lipase in Section III Practical Biochemistry.

CHAPTER

8

Oral Glucose Tolerance Test

Oral glucose tolerance test (OGTT) is the ability to tolerate glucose.

Indications

1. Patient has symtoms suggestive of diabetes mellitus but has inconclusive values of fasting or postprandial blood glucose.
2. To diagnose gestational diabetes mellitus.

Contraindications

1. Known case of diabetes mellitus.
2. Severely ill patients.

Preparation of the Patient

1. Patients should have good carbohydrate diet for three days prior to the test.
2. Drugs affecting blood glucose must be stopped two days prior to the test.
3. Avoid strenuous exercise 1 day prior to the test.
4. Avoid smoking and alcohol during the test.
5. Have dinner at 8 pm on the previous night of the test.

Procedure of the Test

Patient must be in overnight fasting for 10–12 hours after the previous night dinner

↓

Patient must not have breakfast or tea or coffee on the day of the test

↓

Fasting sample of blood and urine collected at 8 am

↓

75 g of glucose dissolved in 200 ml of water is given

↓

Patient must drink it slowly in 5 minutes

↓

Sample of blood and urine collected after 2 hours (2-hour sample)—
2-hour postglucose load

Conventional GTT (extended GTT): 6 samples (0 hr, ½ hr, 1 hr, 1½ hr, 2 hr, 2½ hr).

Modern GTT (mini GTT): 2 samples (0 hr, 2 hr).

IV GTT (intravenous GTT): It is a measure of insulin secretory capacity in response to sudden increase in blood glucose. Not done nowadays.

Glucose challenge test (GCT): Irrespective of feeding status, 50 mg glucose is given oral and blood glucose is checked after 1 hour. 1 hour postglucose load value >140 mg/dL is an indication to do GTT.

Diagnostic Criteria

	Normal	*IGT*	*Diabetes mellitus*
Fasting	<100 mg/dL	100–125 mg/dL	≥126 mg/dL
2 hours	<140 mg/dL	140–199 mg/dL	≥200 mg/dL

Diabetes in Pregnancy Study Group of India (DIPSI)

- Overnight fasting is not required.
- 75 g of glucose is given irrespective of their food intake.
- A blood sample is collected after 2 hours.
- 2 hours value >140 mg/dL is suggestive of gestational diabetes mellitus.

CHAPTER

9

Clinical Enzymology Enzymes Used as Cardiac Markers

Indications

1. Diagnosis of myocardial infarction
2. Recurrent myocardial infarction
3. Serial monitoring in myocardial infarction

Cardiac Marker Enzymes

1. Troponin T and I
   - Most sensitive and specific
   - Commonly used
2. CK-MB
   - Creatinine kinase
   - CK-MB is 5% of CK-total
3. LDH
   - Non-specific
   - Flipped pattern LDH1 > LDH_2 in myocardial infarction
4. Myoglobin
   - Negative marker
5. IMA
   - Ischemia modified albumin
   - Negative marker
6. AST
   - Non-specific
   - Increase in liver disease

Enzyme Kinetics

S. No	*Enzyme*	*Starts*	*Peak*	*Normal in*
1	CK-MB	3–6 hours	24 hours	72 hours
2	Troponin T	6 hours	72 hours	14 days
3	Troponin I	4 hours	24 hours	10 days

Normal Values

1. **CK-MB:** 5–25 IU/L
2. **Troponin T:** 0–0.4 ng/mL
3. **Troponin I:** 1–10 µg/L

Method of Assay

1. Colorimetry
2. ECLIA
3. ELFA
4. POCT devices

CHAPTER

10

Lipid Profile

Tests Under Lipid Profile

1. Serum total cholesterol
2. Serum triglyceride (TG)
3. Serum HDL (high density lipoprotein)
4. Serum VLDL (very low density lipoprotein)
5. Serum LDL (low density lipoprotein)

Indications to do Lipid Profile

1. Cardiac diseases
2. Diabetes mellitus
3. Hypertension
4. Renal disease
5. Thyroid disorders
6. Age >40 years
7. Family history of lipid dysfunction

Sample Required

A fasting blood sample (after 10–12 hours of fasting) is preferred.

Refer to Chapters 9,10, 11 in Practical Biochemistry section on Estimation of Lipid parameters.

Lipid profile	
Total cholesterol	<200 mg/dl
Triglycerides	<150 mg/dl
HDL cholesterol	>40 mg/dl
LDL cholesterol	<100 mg/dl
VLDL cholesterol	<30 mg/dl

CHAPTER

11

Cerebrospinal Fluid Analysis

- CSF—cerebrospinal fluid
- The total volume of CSF is 125 ml
- CSF chloride >plasma chloride

Indications for CSF Analysis

1. Bacterial meningitis
2. Viral meningitis
3. Brain tumors

Laboratory Investigations

1. Appearance—clear and colorless
2. Cell count and cytology
3. CSF protein
   - Microprotein by PGR method
   - Normal level is 10–30 mg/dL
4. CSF glucose
   - GOD–POD method
   - Normal level is 50–70 mg/dL
5. CSF chloride
6. Special investigations
   - CSF ADA for tuberculosis
   - CSF electrophoresis
   - CSF lactate
   - CSF Ig for multiple myeloma

S. No		*Normal*	*Bacterial infection*	*Viral infection*
1	Color	Clear	Turbid	Clear
2	Cell count	$0–4 \times 10^6$/L	↑	↑
3	Protein	10–30 mg/dL	↑↑	↑
4	Glucose	50–70 mg/dL	↓↓	N

CHAPTER

12

Pleural Fluid Analysis

Pleural Effusion

1. Fluid collection in pleural cavity
2. Pleural cavity surrounds lungs
3. Occurs in diseases and cancers
4. Tuberculosis is the common cause
5. Heart disease and dengue also cause pleural effusion

Types

Exudate	Transudate
1. Infection	1. Non inflammatory
2. Purulent	2. Clear
3. Protein >2 g/dL	3. Protein <2 g/dL
4. Specific gravity — High	4. Specific gravity — Low
5. Bacteria –+	5. No bacteria
6. Cell count — High	6. Cell count — Low
7. LDH — High	7. LDH — Low

Light's Criteria for Exudate

1. Pleural fluid/serum protein >0.5
2. Pleural fluid/serum LDH >0.6
3. Pleural fluid LDH >2/3 upper limit of normal

Biochemical Tests

Pleural fluid:

- Protein (microprotein kit)
- Glucose
- ADA for tuberculosis
- LDH

Pathology

Pleural fluid—cytology

Microbiology

Pleural fluid:

- AFB stain
- Gram's stain
- Culture/sensitivity
- PCR

CHAPTER

13

Arterial Blood Gas Analysis

An acid is a chemical that can donate protons.

A base is a chemical that can accept protons.

pH is the negative logarithm of H+ ion concentration.

Buffers

A buffer is a solution that can resist changes in pH when a small quantity of acid or base is added.

The acid–base balance of the body is maintained by:

1. Blood buffers
2. Respiratory mechanism
3. Renal mechanism

Blood Buffer Systems

1. Bicarbonate buffer system
2. Phosphate buffer system
3. Protein buffer system

Respiratory Regulation

When the blood pH decreases, the respiratory rate is increased which eliminates CO_2. Hence pH returns to normal. When the blood pH increases, the respiratory centre is inhibited and CO_2 is retained. Thus pH is returned to normal.

Renal Regulation

The Kidneys regulate acid-base homeostasis by the following mechanisms of:

1. Excretion of H^+ ions
2. Reabsorption of bicarbonate
3. Phosphate mechanism
4. Ammonia excretion

Acid–base Disorders

1. Metabolic acidosis (decrease in pH)

2. Metabolic alkalosis (increase in pH)
3. Respiratory acidosis (excess carbon dioxide)
4. Respiratory alkalosis (CO_2 deficit)

Anion Gap

It is a measure of unmeasured anions.

$$\text{Anion gap} = (Na + K) - (HCO_3 + Cl)$$

Acid–base Analysis

ABG (arterial blood gas analysis) is done using a blood gas analyser that measures pH, pO_2 and pCO_2 using ion-selective electrodes.

Refer to Chapter 11 Arterial Blood Gas Analyser in Section II.

CHAPTER

14

Plasma Proteins

- Blood = Plasma 55% + cells (RBC, WBC, platelets) 45%
- Major plasma proteins—albumin, globulin, fibrinogen
- Reference ranges
  - **Total protein:** 6–8 g/dL
  - **Albumin:** 3.5–5 g/dL
  - **Globulin:** 2.5–3.5 g/dL
  - **A : G ratio:** 1.2:1 to 1.5:1
- Proteins are synthesised in liver
- Calcium-dependent clotting factors—7, 9, 10, 11, 12
- Vitamin K-dependent clotting factors—2, 7, 9, 10
- Plasma proteins are separated by:
  1. Electrophoresis
  2. SDS PAGE
  3. HPLC
  4. Ultracentrifugation

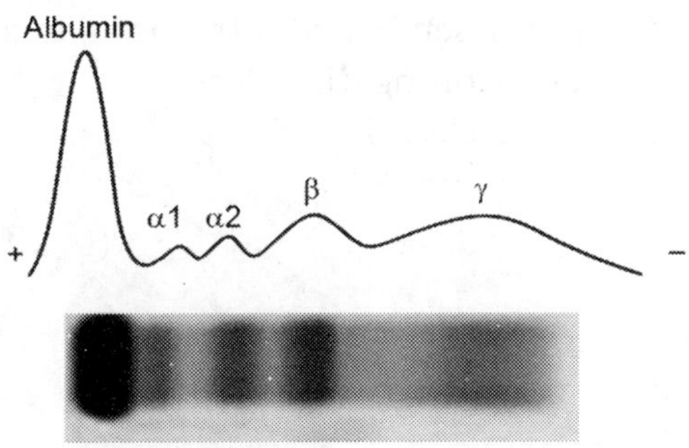

Albumin 55–65%

Globulin
- α_1 — 2 to 4%
- α_2 — 6 to 12%
- β — 8 to 12%
- γ — 12 to 22%

Functions of Plasma Proteins

1. Maintenance of colloid osmotic pressure
2. Maintenance of blood pressure
3. Maintenance of acid–base balance
4. Role in transport
5. Role in immunity
6. Role in inflammation
7. Enzymes
8. Role in blood coagulation

Acute Phase Reactants (APR)—Inflammatory Markers

1. CRP
2. Ferritin
3. Fibrinogen
4. C3, C4
5. Ceruloplasmin
6. Procalcitonin

CHAPTER

15

Fibrinogen

- It is clotting factor 1
- It forms fibrin clot
- It is formed in liver
- Fibrin is insoluble
- It is a acute phase protein
- Normal value is 200–400 mg/dL
- It is a test in coagulation profile
- It can be measured by a semi-automated or fully automated analyzer, e.g. STAGO (STA Compact Max analyser), ECL 90.

Fibrinogen levels are increased in:

1. DIC (disseminated intravascular coagulation)
2. Blood clotting disorders
3. Atherosclerosis.

CHAPTER

16

Prothrombin Time (PT)

- Prothrombin time is the time taken by blood to clot after the addition of calcium and tissue thromboplastin.
- PT measures the extrinsic pathway of coagulation.

Principle

Citrated plasma $\xrightarrow[\text{Calcium}]{\text{Tissue thromboplastin}}$ Activates extrinsic pathways factors → Soild gel clot is formed

- Excess of calcium reverses the effects of citrate
- The time taken to form this solid gel clot is measured

Reagent

Lyophilised calcified thromboplastin from rabbit brain

Preparation

Bring PT reagent to normal temperature

↓

Reconstitute with 4 ml of distilled water

↓

Mix thoroughly before using

Anticoagulant for Sample

3.2% sodium citrate—0.2 ml

+

Blood—1.8 ml

Procedure

- PT is measured using a semi-automated or fully automated analyzer
- Citrated plasma is taken in a cuvette with a metal bead inside it
- On adding the reagent, the stirrer movement of the metal bead stops due to formation of gel clot
- This time is measured optically

INTERNATIONAL NORMALISED RATIO (INR)

$$INR = \left[\frac{PT\ (Test)}{PT\ (Control)}\right]^{ISI}$$

ISI—International sensitivity index
INR helps to compare the prothrombin time (PT) of different labs
Reference range of PT—12 to 15 seconds
Reference range of INR—0.8 to 1.2

PT is increased in:

1. Liver diseases
2. Vitamin K deficiency
3. Patients taking anticoagulants

INR is monitored in:

1. Deep vein thrombosis (DVT)
2. Heart valves surgery
3. Patients taking anticoagulants

CHAPTER

17

Applications of Radioisotopes

Isotopes

They have the same atomic number but different mass number.

Example: $_1H^1$—Hydrogen
$_1H^2$—Deuterium
$_1H^3$—Tritium

Radioactivity

The unstable isotopes that emit rays by spontaneous degradation of its nucleus is called radioactivity.

Commonly Used Radioisotopes

1. Carbon ^{14}C—carbon dating
2. Hydrogen ^{3}H—research
3. Phosphorus ^{32}P—blood cancer treatment
4. Iodine ^{131}I—thyroid treatment

Applications

1. To trace the biochemical pathways
2. To calculate total blood volume
3. Carbon dating
4. Radioimmunoassay
5. Thyroid scan
6. PET scan.

CHAPTER

18

Stone Analysis

FORMATION OF STONES

Kidney stones or renal calculi are made of mineral and acid salts.
Kidney stones may be present in renal pelvis, ureter, urinary bladder or urethra

Types of Renal Stones

1. Calcium oxalate stones
2. Triple phosphate stones (struvite stones)
3. Uric acid stones
4. Cystine stones.

Causes

1. Decreased fluid intake.
2. Increased concentration of calcium, phosphorus, uric acid, oxalate, and cystine.

INVESTIGATIONS FOR RENAL STONES

Sample Collection

- Early morning first void urine
- Urine can be filtered for stones if present

1. **Urine microscopy** to look for RBCs, pus cells and the shape of crystals

   Urine crystals

   a. Calcium oxalate dihydrate—envelope shaped
   b. Calcium oxalate monohydrate—dumbell shaped
   c. Uric acid—rhomboid/parallelogram crystals
   d. Triple phosphate/struvite—coffin lid appearance
   e. Cystine—hexagonal crystals
2. **Urine culture** for infections that can be seen in struvite stones
3. **Stone analysis**

   Qualitative analysis of stone composition
4. **Other biochemical investigations**

   a. Renal function tests
   b. Serum electrolytes
   c. Serum calcium, phosphorus, uric acid
   d. Serum parathormone
5. **24-hour urine** for calcium, phosphorus and uric acid

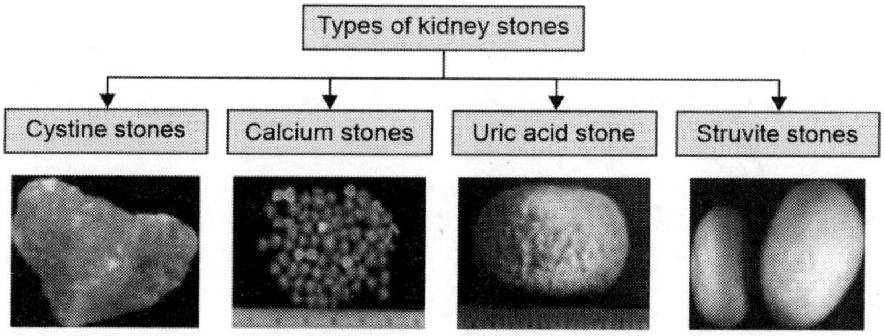

Gross appearance of renal stones

QUALITATIVE ANALYSIS OF RENAL STONES

The stone sample is powdered using a pestle and mortar and a solution is made out of it using dil. HCl.

Experiments	*Observation*	*Inference*
1. Test for uric acid		
Principle: Uric acid is oxidised by HNO_3 to form an orange-colored complex		
Add 5 drops of conc. Nitric acid to 0.5 ml of sample	Yellow to orange colored complex	Presence of uric acid
2. Test for carbonate		
Carbonate reacts with hydrochloric acid to form calcium chloride and carbon dioxide is released		
Add 0.5 ml of dil. Hydrochloric acid to 0.5 ml of sample	Gas bubbles are seen	Presence of carbonate
3. Test for oxalate		
Oxalate reacts with potassium permanganate to form a white precipitate of potassium oxalate		
A part of sample is heated with dil. sulfuric acid and then add 2 drops of potassium permanganate solution and mix	A white precipitate is formed	Presence of oxalate
4. Test for phosphates		
Principle: Phosphate ions react with ammonium molybdate to form a characteristic yellow precipitate of ammonium phosphomolybdate		
To a small amount of sample add 1.5 ml of concentrated nitric acid and 1.5 ml of ammonium molybdate solution and heat	A yellow precipitate is formed	Presence of phosphates
5. Test for calcium		
Principle: Calcium forms a white precipitate of calcium oxalate with ammonium oxalate		
To 1 ml of sample add 1 ml ammonium oxalate	A white precipitate is formed	Presence of calcium

Other Methods

Several methods can be used for analysis of structure and composition of the stones

- Infrared spectroscopy
- Atomic absorption spectroscopy
- Polarization microscopy
- Roentgen-structural analysis

SECTION

V

Metabolism

1. Metabolism of Carbohydrates
2. Metabolism of Lipids
3. Metabolism of Amino Acids and Proteins
4. Hemoglobin Metabolism
5. Neonatal Screening for Inborn Errors of Metabolism, Phenylketonuria, and Albinism
6. Enzymology
7. Obesity

CHAPTER

1

Metabolism of Carbohydrates

CLASSIFICATION OF CARBOHYDRATES

Carbohydrates are polyhydroxy aldehydes or ketones.

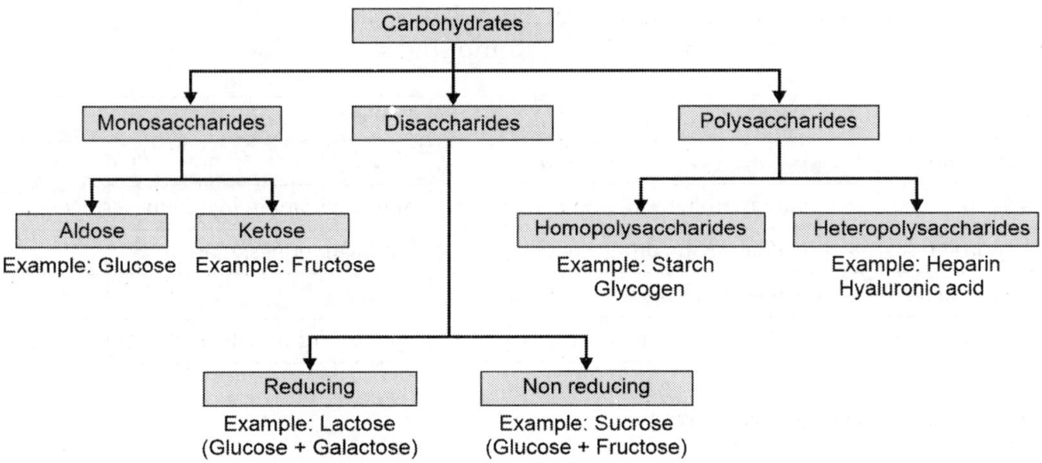

Monosaccharides

- Carbohydrates with only one sugar molecule.
- It is the simplest sugar.

Disaccharides

- Made up of two sugar molecules.
- Two sugars are linked by glycosidic bond.

Trisaccharides

- It contains three sugar molecules.

Example: Trehalose

Oligosaccharides

Made of few sugar molecules.

Polysaccharides

Composed of more than ten monosaccharide units.

Homopolysaccharides

Made of repeating units of same monosaccharides:

Example:
Starch—storage form of energy in plants
Glycogen—storage form of energy in humans and animals
Inulin—used in GFR calculation
Dextran—used as plasma expander

Heteropolysaccharides

These are polysaccharides with more than one type of sugar molecules.

1. Agar and agarose:
   - Agar is obtained from sea weeds
   - Agarose is used as matrix in electrophoresis
2. Mucopolysaccharides:
   - They are called glycosaminoglycans (GAG)
   - They are made up of uronic acid + amino sugars

Mucopolysaccharide	*Repeating Units*	*Tissue Localisation*
Hyaluronic acid	NaGlu + Glucuronic acid	Vitreous humor, synovial fluid
Heparin	Glucosamine + Iduronic acid	Anticoagulant in liver, lungs, spleen
Chondroitin sulphate	NaGal + Glucuronic acid	Cartilage, bones, tendons
Keratan sulphate	NaGlu + Galactose (No uronic acid)	Cornea
Dermatan sulphate	NaGal + Iduronic acid	Skin, blood vessels, heart valves

FUNCTIONS OF CARBOHYDRATES

1. Carbohydrates are the main source of energy to the body
2. Energy produced is 4 kcal/g
3. **Glycogen** is the storage form of energy
4. **Triglycerides** are synthesized from carbohydrates
5. **Glycoproteins** function as hormones
6. **Glycolipids** act as cell receptors
7. **Mucopolysaccharides** are the ground substance in bones, cornea and blood vessels
8. **Blood group antigens** are made up of carbohydrates and amino sugars
9. Glucose is the only source of energy for RBC and the brain
10. **Glycocalyx** are found on the surface of the cell membrane.

Digestion and Absorption of Carbohydrates

Digestion is the breakdown of complex carbohydrates (polysaccharides) into simple carbohydrates (monosaccharides).

$$\text{Starch} \xrightarrow{\text{Amylase}} \text{Dextrins}$$

$$\text{Glycogen} \xrightarrow{\text{Amylase}} \text{Maltose and isomaltose}$$

$$\text{Lactose} \xrightarrow{\text{Lactase}} \text{Glucose} + \text{Galactose}$$

$$\text{Sucrose} \xrightarrow{\text{Sucrase}} \text{Glucose} + \text{Fructose}$$

$$\text{Maltose} \xrightarrow{\text{Maltase}} \text{Glucose}$$

$$\text{Isomaltose} \xrightarrow{\text{Isomaltase}} \text{Glucose}$$

$$\text{Trehalose} \xrightarrow{\text{Trehalase}} \text{Glucose}$$

Glucose Transporters

Glucose transporters (GluT) help in the absorption of glucose.

Transporter	*Location*
GluT 1	RBC
GluT 2	Beta cells of the pancreas, liver
GluT 3	Neurons, brain
GluT 4	Skeletal muscle (insulin-dependent)
GluT 5	Testis (fructose transporter)
SGluT 1	Intestine
SGluT 2	Kidney

Galactosemia

Inborn error of galactose metabolism

Enzyme defect: Galactose-1-phosphate uridyl transferase.

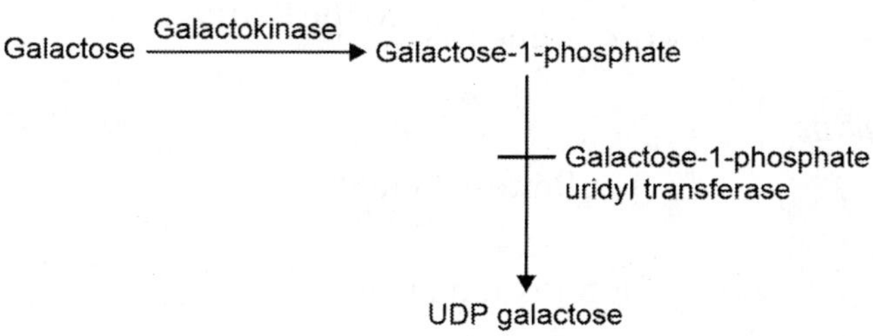

Clinical Manifestations

1. Jaundice—bilirubin uptake is less or bilirubin conjugation is reduced, unconjugated bilirubin level is increased
2. Mental retardation
3. Hypoglycemia
4. Congenital cataract
5. Aminoaciduria.

Diagnosis

1. Mucic acid test
2. Presence of galactose in urine—Benedict's test
3. Elevated blood galactose levels
4. Amniocentesis.

Treatment

Lactose-free diet.

DIABETES MELLITUS

- Diabetes mellitus is a state of hyperglycemia
- It is due to insulin deficiency or insulin resistance.

Types

1. Type 1 diabetes mellitus (T1 DM/IDDM)
2. Type 2 diabetes mellitus (T2 DM/NIDDM)
3. Secondary diabetes mellitus
4. Gestational diabetes mellitus (GDM)

Type 1 Diabetes Mellitus

Beta cells destroyed by auto antibodies

↓

Insulin production is less

↓

Insulin injection is needed

↓

Starts at 11 to 15 years of age

↓

More prone to ketosis

Type 2 Diabetes Mellitus

Insulin resistance

↓

High insulin levels

↓

GLUT 4 failure

↓

High glucose in the blood

↓

Starts >40 years of age

↓

Less prone to ketosis

Diagnosis

1. Interpretation

	Fasting F (mg/dL)	*Post prandial PP (mg/dL)*
Normal	<100	<140
Diabetes mellitus	≥ 126	≥ 200

2. Random blood glucose ≥ 200 mg/dL on two occasions
3. HbA1c $\geq 6.5\%$

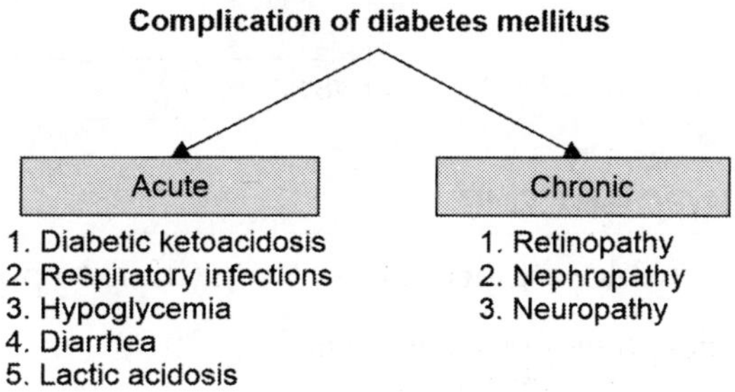

Symptoms

1. Polyphagia
2. Polyuria
3. Polydipsia
4. Infections

Laboratory Diagnosis

1. Blood glucose (grey tube)
2. Urine glucose
3. HbA1c
4. OGTT
5. RFT—urea, creatinine, electrolytes
6. Lipid profile
7. Urine microalbumin
8. Urine ketones.

HBA1c (GLYCATED HEMOGLOBIN)

- Glycated hemoglobin is non-enzymatic addition of glucose to amino group of hemoglobin
- It reflects the glycemic status of an individual over a period of 8 to 12 weeks.

Advantages

- It is used for the diagnosis of diabetes mellitus
- It is used to check the glycemic control following treatment of diabetes mellitus
- It predicts complications of diabetes mellitus
- Fasting sample is not required
- HbA1c is stable
- It is unaffected by day to day glucose fluctuations, exercise or recent food intake

Methods of Estimation

- Immunoturbidimetry method
- HPLC—gold standard method

Interpretation

HbA1c value	*Interpretation*
<5.7%	Normal
5.7–6.4%	Pre-diabetes
>6.5%	Diabetes mellitus
6.5–7%	Adequate control
7–8%	Inadequate control
>8%	Poor control

HYPOGLYCEMIA

Low blood glucose of <60 mg/dL is hypoglycemia.

Symptoms of hypoglycemia:

- Excessive sweating
- Palpitation
- Giddiness
- Loss of consciousness
- Disorientation
- Coma

Causes of hypoglycemia:

- Starvation
- Insulin overdosage
- Chronic alcoholism
- Liver disease
- Glycogen storage disorders (Von Gierke's disease)
- Galactosemia

CHAPTER

2

Metabolism of Lipids

CHOLESTEROL AND BILE SALTS

Cholesterol and its Functions

- Cholesterol is a 27-carbon compound
- It is formed from acetyl CoA by HMG CoA reductase

Types of cholesterol:

Total cholesterol = HDL cholesterol + LDL cholesterol + VLDL cholesterol

- HDL cholesterol—good cholesterol
- LDL cholesterol—atherosclerosis and myocardial infarction risk
- VLDL cholesterol—increased in diabetes mellitus

Regulation of Cholesterol Synthesis

- Cholesterol synthesis is regulated by SREBP and SCAP
- SREBP—sterol regulatory element binding protein
- SCAP—SREBP cleavage activator protein.

Functions of Cholesterol

1. Component of cell membrane
2. Maintains fluidity of cell membrane
3. Nerve conduction
4. Synthesis of steroid hormones (estrogen, progesterone, cortisol, aldosterone), vitamin D, bile salts
5. Esterified with PUFA (polyunsaturated fatty acids) and excreted in liver.

Bile Salts

1. Bile salts are sodium or potassium salts of bile acids
2. Bile acids are 24-carbon compounds
3. Bile acids are formed from cholesterol by 7α hydroxylase
4. Bile salts are excreted in bile
5. Bile salts undergo enterohepatic circulation.

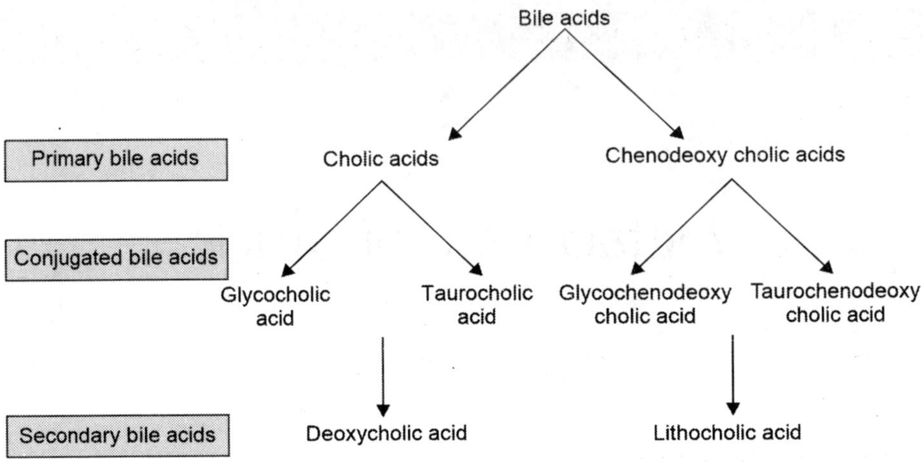

Functions of Bile

1. Absorption of lipids by micelle formation
2. Act as surfactant
3. Neutralise the acidity of gastric juice
4. Excretion of cholesterol and bilirubin
5. Conjugation and detoxification of drugs
6. Nutrient signaling molecule through LXR, FXR.

Atherosclerosis

Atherosclerosis is a degenerative disease of blood vessels resulting in stiffening.

Stages of Atherosclerosis

Stage 1: Formation of foam cells

Stage 2: Fatty streak formation

Stage 3: Early plaque formation

Stage 4: Advanced fibrous plaque and plaque rupture

Four stages of atherosclerosis

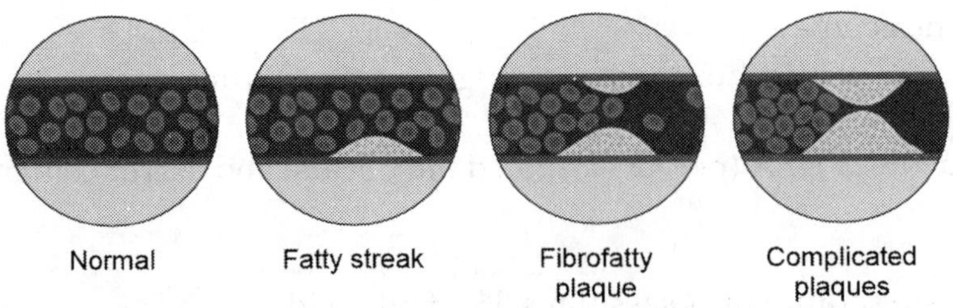

Risk Factors of Atherosclerosis

1. Smoking
2. Alcohol

3. Obesity
4. Hypertension
5. Diabetes mellitus
6. Increased lipoprotein (a)
7. Increased hs-CRP
8. Age
9. Male
10. Family history

Markers of Atherosclerosis

1. Total cholesterol
2. Triglycerides
3. Low HDL
4. Increased LDL, lipoprotein (a)
5. hs-CRP
6. Homocysteine levels
7. AST
8. LDH
9. Apo B: Apo A1 ratio
10. Waist circumference, waist–hip ratio

CLASSIFICATION OF LIPIDS

Based on chemical nature, lipids are classified as:

1. Simple lipids
2. Compound lipids
3. Derived lipids
4. Lipid complexes

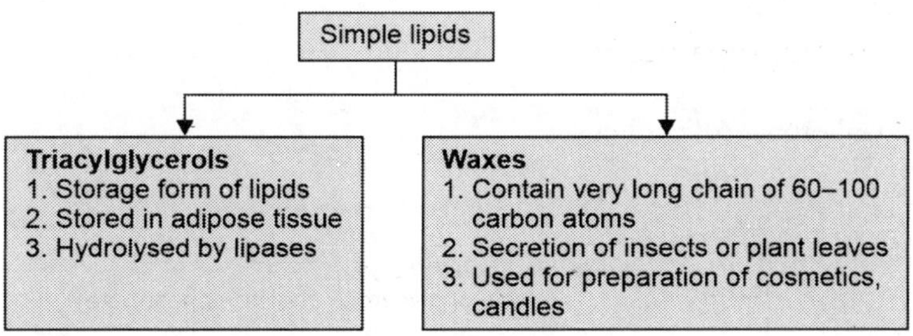

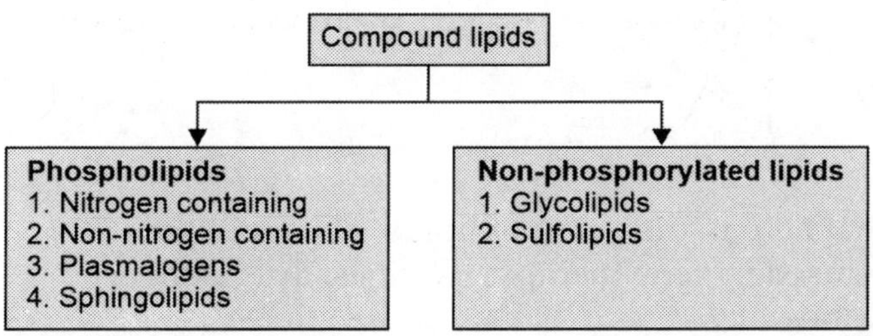

Derived Lipids

1. Derived lipids include the fatty acids
2. Fatty acids are the major lipids of the body
3. Fatty acids + glycerol = triglyceride
4. Free fatty acids are harmful

Types of Fatty acids

1. Even chain fatty acids
   Has even number of carbon atoms
2. Odd chain fatty acids
   Has odd number of carbon atoms
3. Short chain fatty acids
   Has 2 to 6 carbon atoms
4. Medium chain fatty acids
   Has 8 to 14 carbon atoms
5. Long chain fatty acids
   Has 16 to 24 carbon atoms
6. Very long chain fatty acids
   Has more than 24 carbon atoms
7. Saturated fatty acids
   Has no double bond
8. Unsaturated fatty acids
   Contains double bond
9. Trans fatty acids
   Present in packed dairy foods

Phospholipids

Phospholipids contain a phosphoric acid and 2 fatty acids esterified to glycerol and a nitrogenous base.
Phospholipids are amphipathic

Example: Lecithin (phosphatidyl choline)

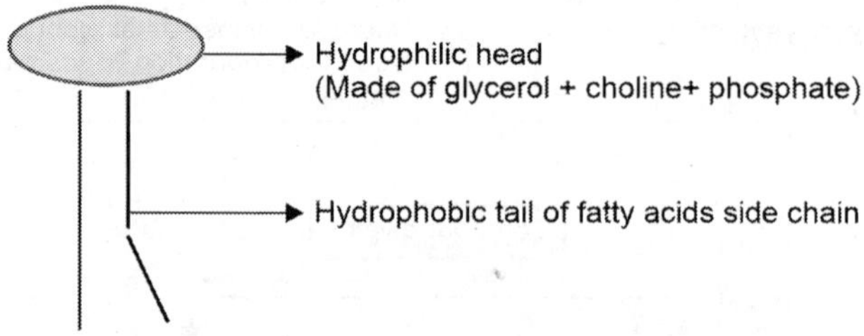

- They can form:
  - Micelles that help in digestion of lipids, phospholipids
  - Liposomes used in gene therapy, vaccines, drug delivery
  - Biomembranes

Phospholipases

Lecithin $\xrightarrow{\text{Phospholipase A2}}$ Lysolecithin + fatty acid (breaks in 2 carbon)

Phospholipase A1 → Removes the fatty acid esterified at 1st carbon

Phospholipase C → Removes the phosphorylcholine at 3rd carbon

Phospholipase D → Removes choline at 3rd carbon

Significance of Phospholipids

1. Phospholipids act as pulmonary surfactants (DPPC and DPL)
2. Deficiency of surfactants leads to:
   - Respiratory distress syndrome
   - Meconium aspiration syndrome
   - Pulmonary alveolar proteinosis
   - Hyaline membrane disease
3. Cephalin is found in cell membranes of brain tissue
4. Phosphatidyl inositol (PIP2) acts a second messenger
5. Plasmalogens are found in cell membranes of brain and muscle
6. Cardiolipin is the phospholipid in mitochondrial membrane of heart
7. Sphingomyelin is abundant in nervous tissue

Classification of Phospholipids

Classification of phospholipids

Nitrogen containing	Non-nitrogen containing	Plasmalogens	Sphingolipids
1. Lecithin 2. Cephalin 3. Phosphatidyl serine	1. Phosphatidyl inositol 2. Phosphatidyl glycerol 3. Cardiolipin	1. Choline plasmalogen 2. Ethanolamine plasmalogen	1. Sphingomyelin

Glycosphingolipids

- They are found in nervous tissue
- They contain ceramide
- They are:
  1. Cerebrosides
  2. Globosides
  3. Gangliosides

Sulfolipids

1. Sulfated cerebrosides
2. Sulfated globosides
3. Sulfated gangliosides

Accumulation of these lipids can lead to lipid storage disorders.

Essential Fatty Acids (EFA)

- Essential fatty acids are polyunsaturated fatty acids
- They are:
    1. Linoleic acid (ω6)
    2. Linolenic acid (ω3)
- They cannot be synthesized in the body and have to be provided in the food

Functions

1. Found in all cell membranes and increases its fluidity
2. They are essential for development of human brain
3. They help in excretion of cholesterol and prevent atherosclerosis
4. They form prostaglandins

Diseases Associated with EFA Deficiency

1. Acanthocytosis, acrodermatitis
2. Atherosclerosis, hypercholesterolemia
3. Retinitis pigmentosa
4. Undergo oxidation by trans-fatty acids and decrease HDL cholesterol levels.

CHAPTER 3

Metabolism of Amino Acids and Proteins

DIGESTION AND ABSORPTION OF PROTEINS

1. Proteins are denatured by cooking
2. Cooking makes the digestion of proteins easy

Dietary proteins
↓ Proteolytic enzymes/peptidases
Dipeptides, tripeptides, amino acids

3. All peptidases are hydrolases
4. All peptidases are inactive zymogens

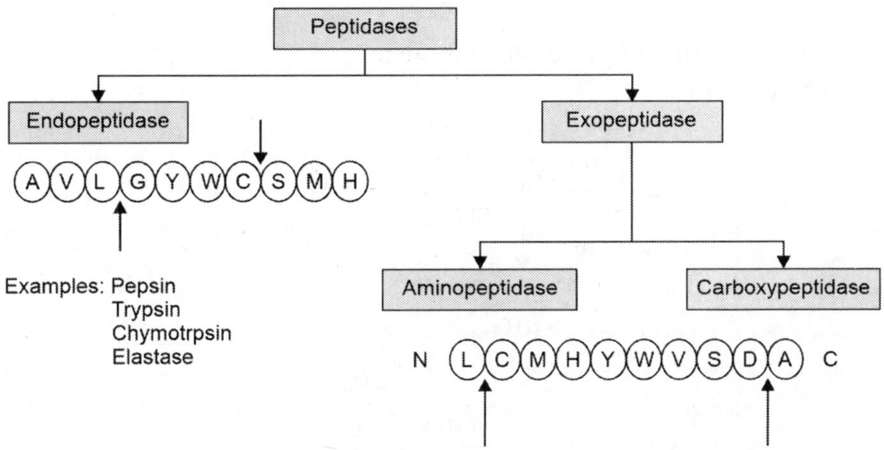

S. No	Inactive enzyme	Active enzyme	Breaking point
1	Pepsinogen	Pepsin	Phe, Tyr, Trp, Met
2	Trypsinogen	Trypsin	Arg, Lys
3	Chymotrypsinogen	Chymotrypsin	Phe, Tyr, Trp, Val, Leu
4	Proelastase	Elastase	Ala, Gly, Ser
5	Procarboxypeptidase	Carboxypeptidase	C terminal amino acid

Absorption of Proteins—Meister Cycle (Gamma Glutamyl Cycle)

Sodium-dependent carrier-mediated transport

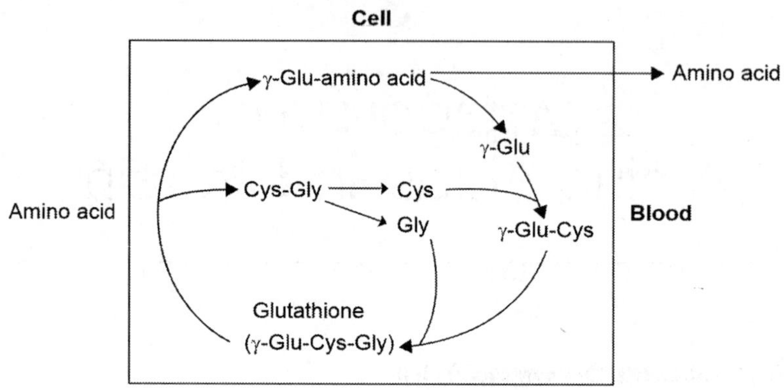

Clinical Conditions

1. Protein malnutrition (kwashiorkor)
2. Protein-losing enteropathy
3. Hartnup's disease
4. Cystinuria
5. Glycinuria

Urea Cycle

- Urea is the end product of protein metabolism.
- Urea is formed in the liver.

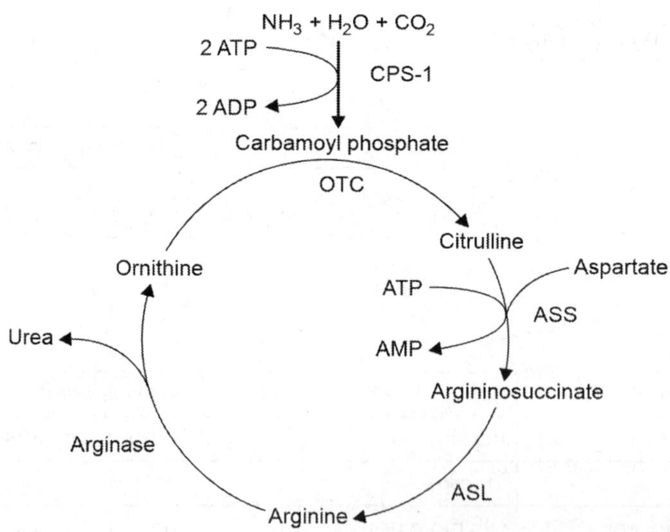

CPS-1: Carbamoyl phosphate synthetase-1
OTC: Ornithine transcarbamylase
ASS: Argininosuccinate synthetase
ASL: Argininosuccinate lyase

Energetics

Used = 4 ATP
1 NADH = 2.5 ATP
Net used = 1.5 ATP

Regulation

1. N acetylglutamate $\xrightarrow{\text{Activates}}$ Carbamoyl phosphate synthetase I.
2. Compartmentalisation.

Clinical Significance

1. Normal blood urea level—15 to 35 mg/dL.
2. Urea is estimated by the urease GLDH method.

STRUCTURAL ORGANISATION OF PROTEINS

LEVELS OF PROTEIN ORGANISATION

1. Primary structure
2. Secondary structure
3. Tertiary structure
4. Quaternary structure

Primary Structure

Primary structure denotes the number and sequence of amino acids in the proteins

- The amino acid sequence is decided by the genes
- Primary structure determines biological activity
- Primary structure is maintained by peptide bonds and disulphide bridges

Example: Insulin has 2 polypeptide chains with 2 inter-chain and 1 intra-chain disulphide bridges

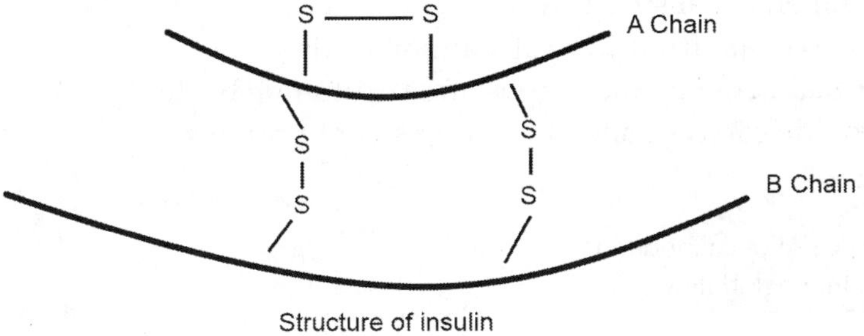

Structure of insulin

Secondary Structure

Secondary structure denotes the steric relationship between amino acids close to each other.

The secondary structure is stabilized by:

- Hydrogen bonds
- Electrostatic bonds

- Hydrophobic interactions
- van der Waals forces

Types of secondary structure

↓ ↓

α Helix
- Most common and stable conformation
- Right-handed helix, e.g. myoglobin

β pleated sheet
- Parallel and antiparallel beta sheets are present, e.g. carbonic anhydrase

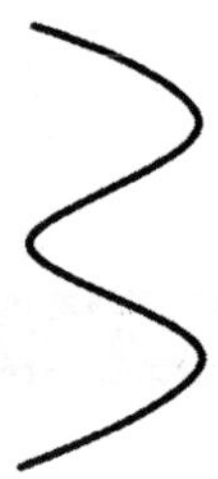

Alpha helix

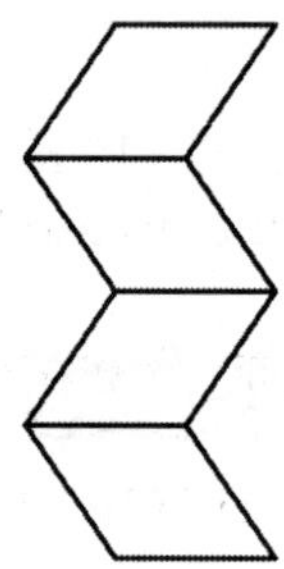

Beta pleated sheets

Tertiary Structure

- Tertiary structure denotes the three-dimensional structure of the whole protein
- It defines the steric relationship of amino acids that are far from each other in primary structure but close to each other in three-dimensional structure
- Tertiary structure is maintained by non-covalent interactions like:
  - Hydrophobic bonds
  - Electrostatic bonds
  - van der Waals forces

Domain

- It is the functional unit of a protein
- It is a three-dimensional structure
- Domains may contain from 25 to 500 amino acids
- Domains are stabilized by metal ions and disulphide bridges
- Domains provide catalytic site or binding site of proteins

Example:
1. Calcium binding site of calmodulin
2. Domains of immunoglobulins

Motif

- Structural motif is a superstructure found in proteins.
- Types of motifs as shown in figure:
  a. Beta hairpin
  b. Helix loop helix
  c. Zinc finger
  d. Helix turn helix

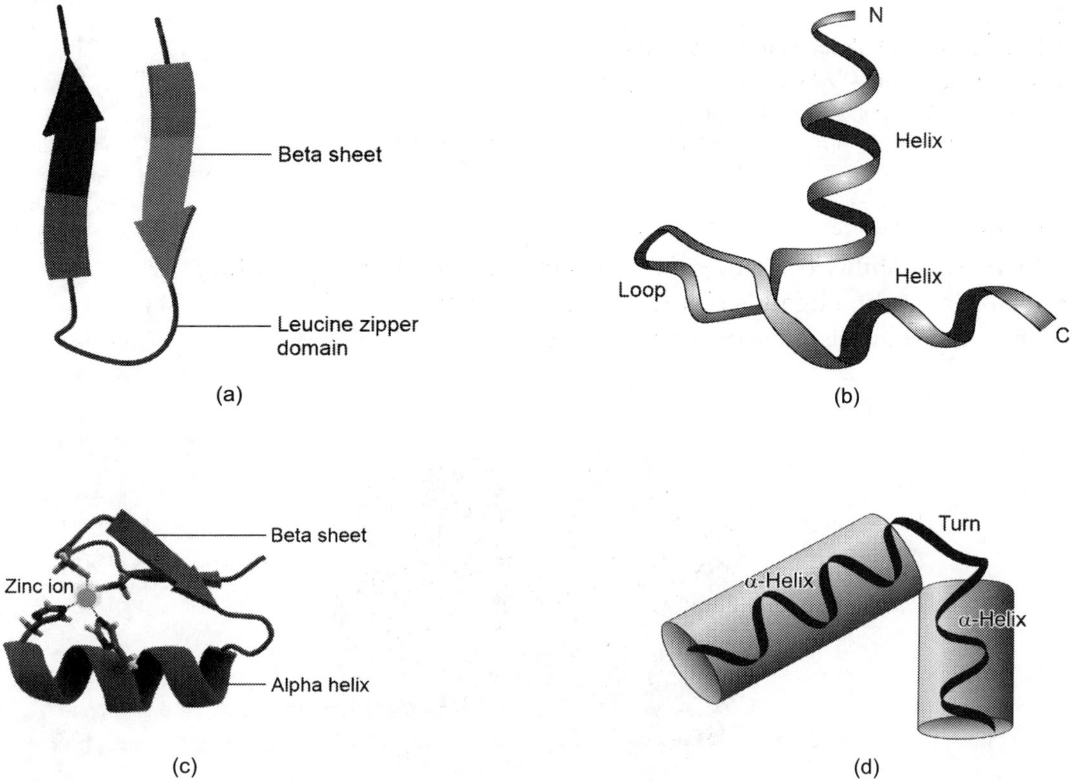

Folds

- Folds are large patterns of the three-dimensional structure of a protein.
- Each fold is associated with a characteristic activity.

> **Example:**
> 1. Actin fold
> 2. Nucleotide-binding fold

Quaternary Structure

- It is the association of individual polypeptide chains to form a functional protein
- Each polypeptide chain is a subunit or monomer
- Homodimer has similar polypeptide chains
- Heterodimer has different polypeptide chains
- Quaternary structure is stabilized by:
  - Hydrogen bonds
  - Electrostatic bonds
  - Hydrophobic bonds
  - van der Waals bonds.

Example:
1. Hemoglobin—2 alpha chains, 2 beta chains.
2. Immunoglobulins—2 heavy chains, 2 light chains.
3. F—actin-oligomer of G—actin subunits.
4. Loss of quaternary structure results in loss of function of protein.

Quaternary structure

- Increases stability of a protein by preventing unfolding or refolding.
- Helps in binding ligands by exhibiting co-operativity.
- Different subunits have different activity.

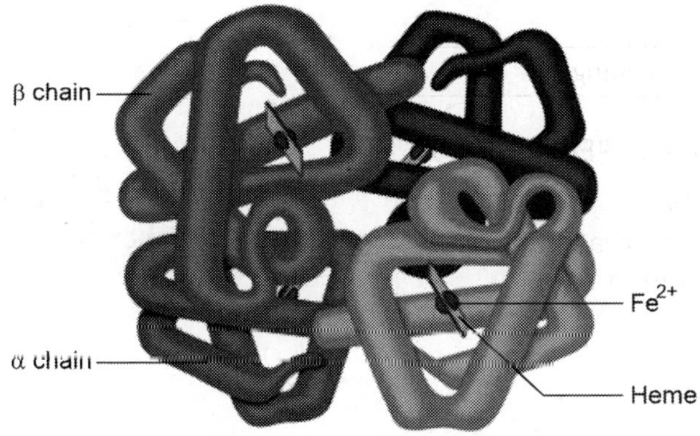

Denaturation

- Loss of quaternary, tertiary and secondary structure of a protein by various agents is called denaturation.
- Primary structure is not altered in denaturation.
- Denaturation results in loss of biological activity of a protein.
- Denaturation can be reversible or irreversible.

Example: Reversible denaturation of immunoglobulin by urea, irreversible denaturation of albumin by heat.

Agents of denaturation

1. pH, heat, high pressure, vigorous shaking.
2. Urea, SDS
3. Advanced glycation end products (AGEs).

Protein Energy Malnutrition (PEM)

PEM is classified into two types:

1. Marasmus—calorie and protein deficiency
2. Kwashiorkor—protein deficiency.

S. No	Marasmus	Kwashiorkor
1.	Less than one year child is affected	It affects 1–5 years of age
2.	Mainly calorie deficiency	Mainly protein deficiency
3.	Child looks very thin and dehydrated	The child looks plumpy due to swollen limbs and abdomen
4.	Skin is dry	Crazy pavement dermatitis
5.	No hair change	Sparse soft hair
6.	Normal appetite	Anorexia present
7.	Watery diarrhoea present	Angular stomatitis present
8.	Albumin 2–3 g/dL	Albumin <2 g/dL
9.	Cortisol is increased	Cortisol is decreased
10.	No fatty liver	Fatty liver is seen
11.	It is due to early weaning	It is due to inadequate protein in the diet

Biochemical Changes in PEM

1. Hypoalbuminemia
2. Fatty liver due to decreased lipoproteins
3. Ig G levels increased
4. Hypoglycemia
5. Hypokalemia
6. Hypomagnesemia
7. Dehydration
8. Vitamin deficiencies.

Treatment of PEM

1. Diet 150–200 kcal/kg body weight
2. 3–4 gm of protein/kg body weight
3. Three parts of vegetable proteins and one part of milk.

Important Compounds Formed from Amino Acids

Amino acid	Important compounds formed
Tyrosine	Melanin, dopamine, nor-epinephrine, epinephrine, thyroxine
Tryptophan	Niacin, serotonin, melatonin
Glycine	Creatinine, heme, purine, glutathione, bile salt
Cysteine	Taurine, glutathione
Arginine	Nitric oxide
Histidine	Histamine

CHAPTER

4

Hemoglobin Metabolism

HEME DEGRADATION

Heme degradation involves the breakdown of heme into bilirubin, which is then transported by albumin and ultimately excreted. Heme breakdown primarily takes place in the spleen.

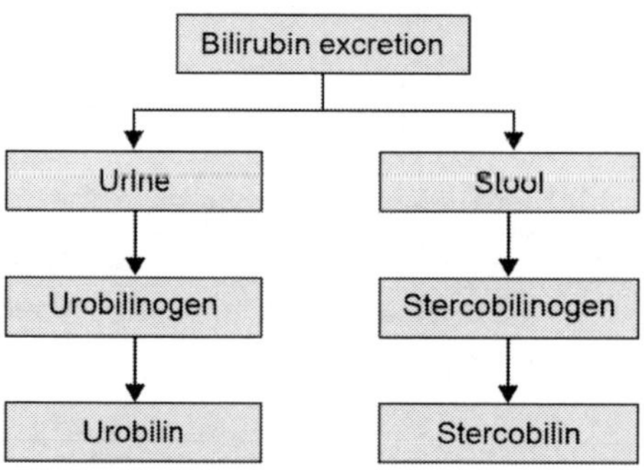

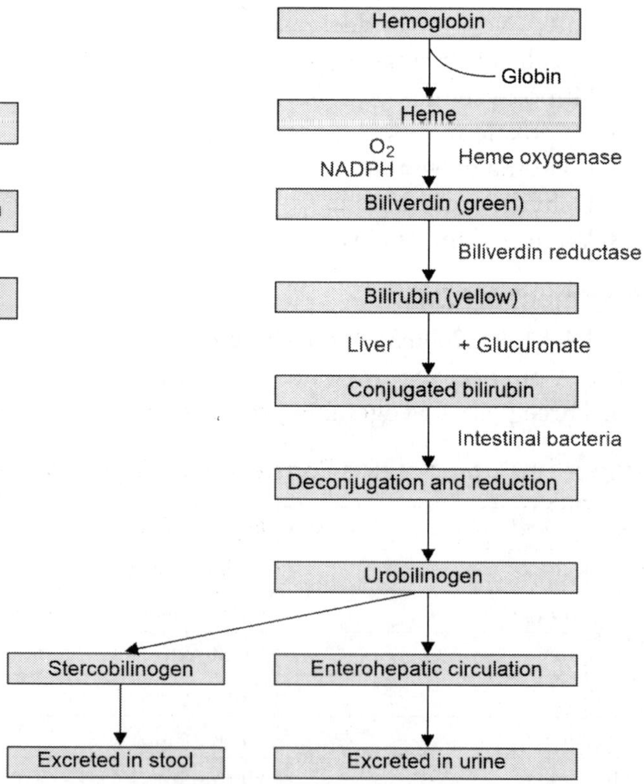

CHAPTER

5 Neonatal Screening for Inborn Errors of Metabolism, Phenylketonuria and Albinism

INBORN ERROR OF METABOLISM (IEM)

Genetic disorders due to defects in metabolism.

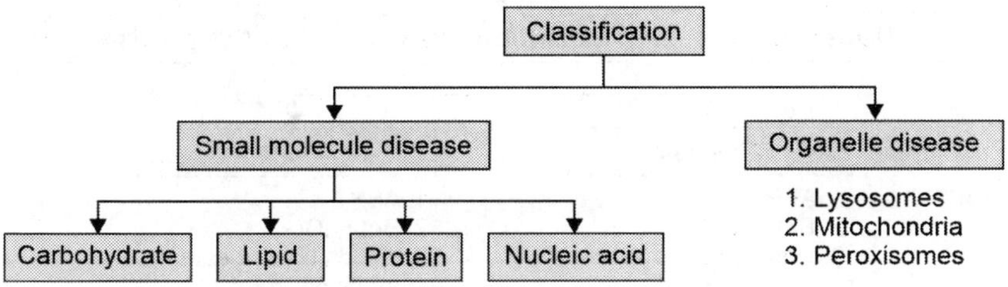

INITIAL LABORATORY SCREENING

Blood

1. Cell count
2. Glucose and ketones
3. Electrolytes
4. Ammonia
5. Uric acid
6. Blood gas analysis (ABG)

Urine

1. Smell
2. pH
3. Ketones, reducing substances

CSF

1. Lactate
2. Pyruvate
3. Glucose

SPECIALIZED BIOCHEMICAL TESTING

1. HPLC: High-performance liquid chromatography
2. Amino acid analysis (plasma and urine)
3. Urine organic acids

GOLD STANDARD TEST FOR DIAGNOSIS OF IEM

Tandem mass spectrometry.

Urine Metabolic Screening Tests

S. No	*Test*	*Observation*	*Inference*
1	Benedict's test	Green/orange/red	Reducing substance
2	Cetrimide test	Cloudy precipitate	Mucopolysaccharides
3	Cyanide nitroprusside test	Pink-red	Cystine, homocysteine
4	DNPH test	Yellow precipitate	PKU, MSUD
5	Ferric chloride test	Green	PKU, MSUD, alkaptonuria

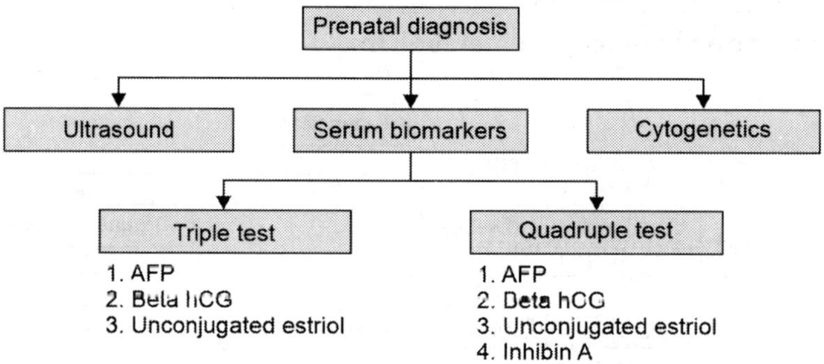

PHENYLKETONURIA

- Phenylketonuria is due to a defect in phenylalanine metabolism.
- It is due to a deficiency of the enzyme phenylalanine hydroxylase.

$$\text{Phenylalanine} \xrightarrow{\text{Phenylalanine hydroxylase}} \text{Tyrosine}$$

Phenylalanine hydroxylase deficiency

↓

Phenylalanine cannot be converted to tyrosine

↓

Phenylalanine accumulates in blood

↓

Phenylalanine converted to phenyl ketones

↓

Phenylketone excreted in urine

Clinical Manifestations

1. Mental retardation
2. Convulsions
3. Hypopigmentation
4. Mousy body odour

Laboratory Diagnosis

1. Guthrie test
2. Ferric chloride test
3. Tandem mass spectrometry
4. DNA probes

Treatment

- Diet containing low phenylalanine
- Tyrosine supplementation

ALKAPTONURIA

- Alkaptonuria is a defect in tyrosine metabolism
- It is due to the deficiency of the enzyme **homogentisate oxidase**

Clinical Manifestations

Homogentisic acid excreted in urine

↓

Urine turns black on exposed to air

↓

In the body, homogentisic acid is oxidized to benzoquinone acetate

↓

Polymerized to black alkapton bodies

↓

Deposited in intervertebral disc, cartilage of nose and ears

↓

Ochronosis

Laboratory Diagnosis

1. Black urine when exposed to air or alkali
2. Ferric chloride test
3. Benedict's test
4. Tandem mass spectrometry

Treatment

A diet containing low phenylalanine.

ALBINISM

1. Albinism is a defect in tyrosine metabolism
2. It is due to deficiency of tyrosinase

$$\text{Tyrosine} \xrightarrow{\text{Tyrosinase}} \text{Melanin (black pigment)}$$

Clinical Manifestations

1. Decreased melanin synthesis
2. Hypopigmented iris

3. Hypopigmented ocular fundus
4. Photophobia
5. Nystagmus
6. Decreased vision
7. Decreased pigmentation of skin
8. Skin is sensitive to UV rays-nevi, melanomas
9. White hair

Laboratory Diagnosis

1. Ferric chloride test
2. Tandem mass spectrometry

Treatment

1. Avoid UV light
2. Sunscreen

INBORN ERRORS OF CARBOHYDRATES METABOLISM

Disorder	*Enzyme deficiency*	*Clinical/lab features*
Pyruvate kinase deficiency	Pyruvate kinase	Hemolytic anemia
von Gierke's disease	Glucose-6-phosphatase	Liver cells and renal tubule cells loaded with glycogen. Hypoglycemia, lactic acidemia, ketosis, hyperlipidemia
Pompe's disease	Acid maltase	Accumulation of glycogen in lysosomes, heart failure, fatal
Forbes' disease or Cori's disease	Debranching enzyme	Accumulation of a characteristic branched polysaccharide
Andersen's disease	Branching enzyme	Accumulation of a polysaccharide having few branch points. Death due to cardiac or liver failure in first year of life
McArdle's syndrome	Muscle phosphorylase	Diminished exercise tolerance; muscles have abnormally high glycogen content (2.5–4.1%). Little or no lactate in blood after exercise
Hers' disease	Liver phosphorylase	High glycogen content in liver, tendency towards hypoglycemia
Tarui's disease	Phosphofructokinase muscle and erythrocytes	Diminished exercise tolerance; muscles have abnormally high glycogen content. Little or no lactate in blood after exercise. Hemolytic anemia
Glucose-6-phosphate dehydrogenase deficiency	Glucose-6-phosphate dehydrogenase	Hemolytic anemia when susceptible individuals are subjected to oxidants
Essential pentosuria	L-xylulose reductase	L-xylulose appears in the urine

Contd...

Disorder	Enzyme deficiency	Clinical/lab features
Hereditary fructose intolerance	Aldolase B	Hypoglycemia accompanied by nausea, vomiting and convulsions
Essential fructosuria	Hepatic fructokinase	A benign condition, as fructose cannot be broken down, so it is simply excreted in the urine
Galactosemia	Galactokinase, uridyl transferase or 4-epimerase	Cataract, liver failure and mental deterioration
Mucopolysaccharidoses	Polysaccharide metabolizing enzymes	Cloudy corneas, mental retardation, stiff joints, cardiac abnormalities, hepatosplenomegaly and short stature. Urine cetrimide test +ve

INBORN ERRORS OF PROTEIN METABOLISM

Disorder	Enzyme deficiency	Clinical/lab features
Hyperammonemia type 1	Carbamoyl phosphate synthetase I	Tremors, slurring of speech, cerebral edema, blurring vision
Hyperammonemia type 2	Ornithine Transcarbamylase	X–linked, glutamine is elevated in blood, cerebrospinal fluid, and urine
Citrullinemia	Argininosuccinate synthase	Tremors, slurring of speech, cerebral edema, blurring vision
Argininosuccinic aciduria	Argininosuccinate lyase	Elevated levels of argininosuccinate in blood, cerebrospinal fluid, and urine. (Trichorrhexis nodosa)
Classical phenylketonuria	Phenylalanine hydroxylase	Seizures, microcephaly, hypopigmentation. Elevated blood Phe levels
Type I Tyrosinemia (Tyrosinosis)	Fumarylacetoacetate hydrolase	Liver failure, increased risk of liver carcinoma, alternate metabolites of tyrosine are also excreted, urine succinyl acetone +ve
Type II Tyrosinemia (Richner-Hanhart syndrome)	Tyrosine aminotransferase	Alternate metabolites of tyrosine are also excreted
Alkaptonuria	Homogentisate oxidase	Urine darkens on exposure to air, arthritis and connective tissue pigmentation (ochronosis)
Xanthurenic Aciduria	Vitamin B_6 deficiency	Excretion of xanthurenate in response to a tryptophan load.
Maple syrup urine disease (Branched-chain ketonuria)	Branched-chain ketoacid Dehydrogenase complex	Burnt sugar odor of urine. Plasma and urinary levels of leucine, isoleucine, valine, α-keto acids, and α-hydroxy acids (reduced α-keto acids) are elevated.
Isovaleric acidemia	Isovaleryl CoA dehydrogenase	Distinctive odor of sweaty feet due to buildup of isovaleric acid. Poor feeding, vomiting, seizures, coma. Plasma also shows hyperammonemia and hyperglycinemia.

INBORN ERRORS OF HEME METABOLISM

Disorder	*Enzyme deficiency*	*Clinical/lab features*	*Special tests*
X-linked sideroblastic anemia	ALA synthase	Anemia, red cell counts and hemoglobin decreased	–
ALA dehydratase deficiency	ALA dehydratase	Abdominal pain, neuropsychiatric symptoms	Urinary aminolevulinic acid
Acute intermittent porphyria	Uroporphyrinogen I synthase	Abdominal pain, neuropsychiatric symptoms	Urinary porphobilinogen positive, uroporphyrin positive
Congenital erythropoietic porphyria	Uroporphyrinogen III synthase	No photosensitivity	Uroporphyrin positive, porphobilinogen negative
Porphyria cutanea tarda	Uroporphyrinogen decarboxylase	Photosensitivity	Uroporphyrin positive, porphobilinogen negative
Hereditary coproporphyria	Coproporphyrinogen oxidase	Photosensitivity, abdominal pain neuropsychiatric symptoms	Urinary porphobilinogen positive, urinary uroporphyrin positive, fecal protoporphyrin positive
Variegate porphyria	Protoporphyrinogen oxidase	Photosensitivity, abdominal pain, neuropsychiatric symptoms	Urinary porphobilinogen positive, fecal protoporphyrin positive
Protoporphyria	Ferrochelatase	Photosensitivity.	Fecal protoporphyrin positive, red cell protoporphyrin positive

CHAPTER

6

Enzymology

CLASSIFICATION OF ENZYMES

Class 1: Oxidoreductases

Help in oxidation-reduction reactions, e.g. alcohol dehydrogenase.

Class 2: Transferases

Help in transfer of groups, e.g. hexokinase, aminotransferase.

Class 3: Hydrolases

Help in hydrolysis, e.g. acetylcholine esterase.

Class 4: Lyase

Help in breaking bonds, e.g. aldolase.

Class 5: Isomerases

Help in forming isomers e.g. isomerase, mutase, racemase.

Class 6: Ligases

Help to link two substrates using ATP, e.g. acetyl CoA carboxylase.

Class 7: Translocases

Transfer of molecules across membrane, e.g. ATP-ADP translocase.

Isoenzymes

- Isoenzymes are different forms of the same enzyme.
- They have different structures but have similar functions.

Types of Isoenzymes

1. True isoenzymes
   Enzymes formed from different genes, e.g. salivary amylase and pancreatic amylase
2. Enzymes with different forms

Example: LDH 1, 2, 3, 4, 5

3. Enzymes located in different tissues

Example: ALP—Alpha 1 (liver)
- Alpha 2 (placenta)
- Pre-beta (bone disease)

4. Enzymes from different alleles of the same gene locus

Example: 400 forms of G6PD

5. Isoforms—due to variations in post-translational modifications

Example: ALP

Identification of isoenzymes

1. Electrophoresis
   Separate isoenzymes with different mobilities
2. Heat stability
3. Inhibitor

Example: Tartrate labile ACP

4. Substrate specificity

Example: Glucokinase—high km
Hexokinase—low km

5. Cofactor requirement
6. Tissue localization

Example: LDH 1 (Heart)
LDH 5 (Skeletal muscle)

7. Specific antibodies.

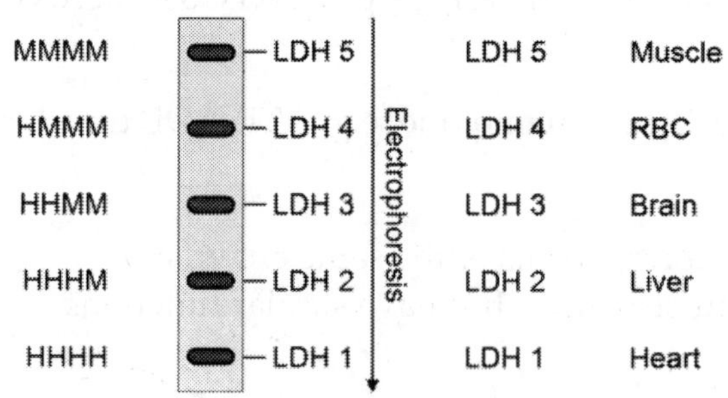

LDH electrophoresis

Coenzymes

1. The non-protein part of the enzyme is called prosthetic part or coenzyme
2. Protein part of the enzyme is the apoenzyme
3. Enzyme = Apoenzyme + Coenzyme

4. Coenzymes are involved in transfer of groups in a chemical reaction
5. Same coenzyme can be shuttled between two reactions helping in coupling of reactions
6. The active form of vitamins and metal ions can function as coenzymes
7. Cofactors include coenzyme and metal ions

Types

- **Coenzymes that transfer hydrogen**
  Example: NAD
  NADP
  FAD
- **Coenzymes that transfer groups other than hydrogen**
  Example: TPP
  PLP
  THFA
- **Metalloenzymes**
  Example: Zn–carbonic anhydrase
  Cu–tyrosinase
  Iron–cytochrome oxidase
  Ca–lipase
  Mo–xanthine oxidase

Example:

Lactate → Pyruvate

NAD^+ → $NADH + H^+$

Alanine + α ketoglutarate → Pyruvate + glutamate

FACTORS AFFECTING ENZYME ACTIVITY

1. Enzyme concentration
2. Substrate concentration
3. Product concentration
4. Effect of temperature
5. Effect of pH
6. Enzyme activation
7. Enzyme inhibition

ENZYME CONCENTRATION

- Rate of a reaction is called velocity (V) of the reaction
- Velocity increases with enzyme concentration

$$\text{Rate of reaction} \propto \text{enzyme concentration}$$

EFFECT OF SUBSTRATE CONCENTRATION

- If substrate concentration is increased, velocity increases initially, then the curve flattens.
- The substrate concentration at which the velocity is half maximum is called K_m
- Maximum velocity is called V_{max}.

Michaelis constant: (K_m)

- K_m is constant for an enzyme
- It is a characteristic feature of an enzyme for a given substrate.
- K_m is not dependent on enzyme concentration
- K_m denotes affinity of an enzyme for substrate

$$K_m \propto \frac{1}{\text{affinity}}$$

Low K_m = high affinity
High K_m = low affinity

Cooperative Binding

Binding of one substrate molecule increases the affinity of binding to other molecules.

EFFECT OF PRODUCT CONCENTRATION

If product concentration increases, reaction slows/stops/reverses.

EFFECT OF TEMPERATURE

- Increase in temperature, increases the velocity initially, reaches a maximum and then decreases.
- The temperature at which the velocity is maximum is called optimum temperature.

Example: Thermus aquaticus has an optimum temperature of 100°C.

EFFECT OF pH

- The activity of an enzyme is maximum at optimum pH.
- Enzymes are inactive at pH lesser than or greater than optimum pH.
- Optimum pH of pepsin is 1–2
- Optimum pH of alkaline phosphatase is 9–10

ENZYME ACTIVATION

Enzymes can be activated by:

1. Inorganic ions

Example: Cl^- activate salivary amylase
Ca^{2+} ions activate lipases

2. Conversion of proenzymes to active enzymes

Example: Trypsinogen = Trypsin
Prothrombin = Thrombin

3. Allosteric activation

ENZYME INHIBITION

Types of Enzyme Inhibition

1. Competitive inhibition
2. Non-competitive inhibition
3. Uncompetitive inhibition
4. Suicidal inhibition
5. Feedback inhibition

COMPETITIVE INHIBITION

- The inhibitor resembles substrate of the enzyme (enzyme analog)
- Inhibitor competes with the substrate to bind to the enzyme.
- Competitive Inhibition is reversible.
- If substrate concentration is increased, inhibition is removed from the enzyme
- In competitive inhibition
  - K_m is increased
  - V_{max} is constant

Example:
1. Xanthine oxidase—allopurinol
2. HMG CoA reductase—statins
3. Dihydrofolate reductase—methotrexate

NONCOMPETITIVE INHIBITION

- The inhibitor does not resemble substrate of the enzyme.
- The inhibitor does not bind to the substrate binding site.
- Inhibitor binds to a separate site. So there is no competition between substrate and Inhibitor.
- Non-competitive inhibition is irreversible.
- In non-competitive inhibition.
  - K_m is constant
  - V_{max} is decreased

Example: Poisons act by non-competitive inhibition

- Cyanide inhibits cytochrome oxidase

UNCOMPETITIVE INHIBITION

- Inhibitor binds to enzyme substrate complex.
- Inhibitor does not bind to free enzyme

$$E + S \rightarrow E - S + I \rightarrow E - S - I$$

- In uncompetitive inhibition
  - K_m is decreased
  - V_{max} is decreased

Example:
- Anticonvulsant valproate
- Phenylalanine inhibiting placental alkaline phosphatase

SUICIDAL INHIBITION

- It is also called mechanism based inactivation.
- It is irreversible.
- The inhibitor is activated by the same enzyme that is inhibited by the activated inhibitor.

Example:
- Allopurinol inhibiting xanthine oxidase
- Aspirin inhibiting cyclooxygenase

FEEDBACK INHIBITION

- The product of the enzyme inhibits the enzyme activity
- It is also known as end product inhibition.
- It happens in biosynthetic pathways to prevent unnecessary product accumulation and wastage of energy.

Example:
- Hexokinase inhibited by glucose-6-phosphate
- ALA synthase inhibited by heme.

CHAPTER

7

Obesity

Obesity is a type of malnutrition where the body mass index (BMI) of an individual is more than 30.

$$\text{Body mass index (BMI)} = \frac{\text{Weight in kg}}{\text{Height in m}^2}$$

Obesity is the result of increased energy consumption with decreased energy utilization.

Causes of Obesity

1. Food habits
2. Lack of exercise
3. Hyperplasia of adipocytes
4. Hypertrophy of adipocytes
5. Genetic factors

Diseases Related to Obesity

1. Decreased insulin sensitivity—diabetes mellitus
2. Metabolic syndrome
   - Hyperglycemia
   - Hyperlipidemia
   - Increased waist–hip ratio
3. Cardiovascular diseases
   - Hypertension
   - Coronary artery disease

Management of Obesity

1. Lifestyle modification
   - Decrease intake of calories and fat
   - Frequent small meals
   - Increase intake of dietary fibres
2. Regular physical activity
   - Helps weight reduction

- Helps weight maintenance
- Yoga and aerobic exercises can also be followed

3. Special diet
   - Atkin's diet [low carbohydrate high protein diet]
   - DASH diet [low-fat diet]
   - Mediterranean diet [fibre-rich diet]
   - Intermittent fasting.
4. Bariatric surgery
   - Gastric banding
   - Gastric bypass

SECTION

VI

Nutrition

CHAPTER

1

Dietary Fibres

Dietary fibres are carbohydrates that are not available for digestion, meaning they are indigestible. The recommended dietary allowance (RDA) for fibre is 30 grams per day. Fruits and vegetables are primary sources of dietary fibre.

Benefits of consuming dietary fibre include:

1. Improving bowel motility
2. Preventing constipation
3. Decreasing cholesterol levels
4. Reducing glucose absorption
5. Lowering the risk of colon cancer
6. Playing an antioxidant role
7. Aiding in weight reduction
8. Preventing inflammatory bowel disease.

Examples of dietary fibres include:

1. Cellulose
2. Hemicellulose
3. Lignin
4. Pectin.

CHAPTER

2

Balanced Diet, BMR, SDA

BALANCED DIET

A balanced diet should contain calories from carbohydrates, proteins and fat in the ratio of 60:20:20.

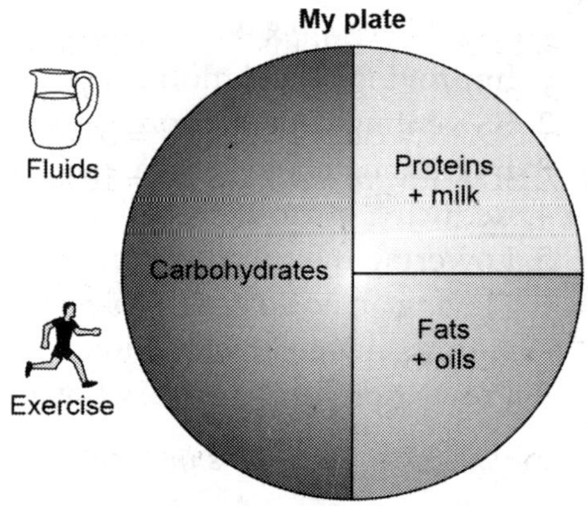

Carbohydrates

- Major energy source.
- 60–65% of total calories.
- Provide dietary fibre.

Proteins

- Building blocks of body tissues.
- 10–15% of total energy.
- Daily requirement for adults—1 g/kg.

Fats

- High energy source.
- 15–20% of total energy.
- 20 g of oils per day, <250 mg/day of cholesterol.
- PUFA, MUFA in 1:1 ratio.

Fluids

- No added sugar/beverages.
- Milk/juices.

Exercise

- Adequate physical activity.

BASAL METABOLIC RATE (BMR)

BMR is the energy required for basal functions like the working of the heart, brain function, respiration, etc. The normal value of BMR in adults is 24 kcal/kg.

Factors Affecting BMR

1. **Age:** BMR is high in active growing age.
2. **Gender:** Males have a higher BMR than females.

3. **Temperature:** BMR increases in cold climate.
4. **Exercise:** BMR is increased.
5. **Fever:** BMR is increased in fever.
6. **Thyroid hormones:** T4 increases BMR.

SPECIFIC DYNAMIC ACTION (SDA)

1. SDA is the heat produced during the digestion of food
2. SDA is the activation energy needed for digestion of nutrients
3. SDA is approximately 10% of the total energy requirement

Example:

Energy requirement	= 1000 kcal
DA	= 10%
10% of 1000	= 100 kcal
Total calories supplied	= 1000 + 100
	= 1100 kcal

4. SDA for proteins = 30%
5. SDA for lipids = 15%
6. SDA for carbohydrates = 5%
7. SDA for mixed food = 10%

CHAPTER

3

Fat Soluble Vitamins

VITAMIN A

Active Forms

- Retinol
- Retinoic acid

Sources

1. Milk
2. Egg yolk
3. Liver
4. Fish liver oil
5. Carrot
6. Papaya
7. Mango
8. Green leafy vegetables

Absorption: Occurs in the small intestine with the assistance of bile salts.

Transport: Facilitated by retinol binding protein (RBP).

Biochemical Functions

1. Wald's visual cycle
2. Dark adaptation—aiding in dim vision
3. Gene regulation—involving RXR, RAR
4. Immunity
5. Reproduction
6. Antioxidant properties
7. Effects on skin

Deficiency Manifestations

1. Night blindness
2. Dry eyes
3. Acne
4. Dry skin

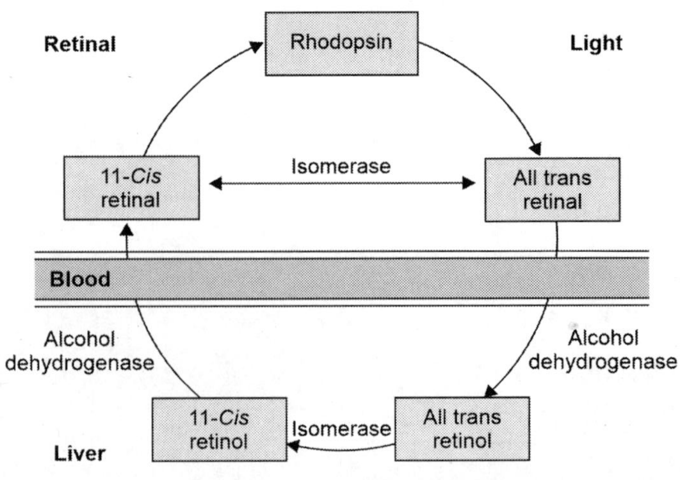

VITAMIN D

Active form: Calcitriol

Formation

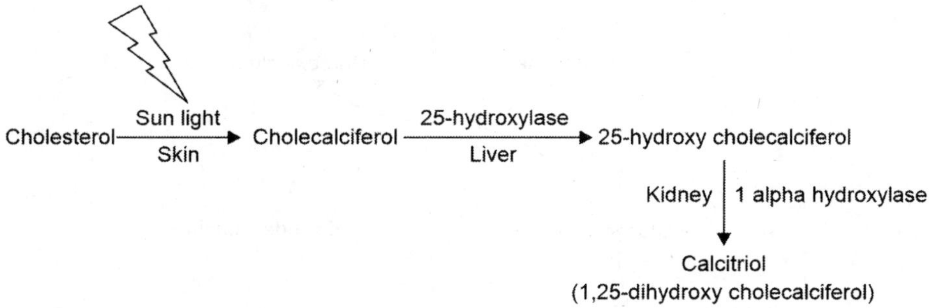

Sources

1. Fish liver oil
2. Fish
3. Egg yolk

Biochemical Functions

1. Calcium absorption
2. Bone mineralization
3. Immunity
4. Prevent GDM, anemia, infections, stroke, cancer, fractures.

Deficiency Disorders

1. Rickets in children
2. Osteomalacia (soft bones) in adults.

VITAMIN K

Vitamin K_1—Phylloquinone
Vitamin K_2—Menaquinone

Sources

1. Green leafy vegetables
2. Intestinal bacteria

Absorption

Small intestine with the help of bile salts.

Storage

Liver

Biochemical Role

1. Blood clotting.
2. Activation of clotting factors 2, 7, 9, 10.

3. Activation of bone protein osteocalcin.
4. Gamma carboxylation of proteins.

Vitamin K Cycle

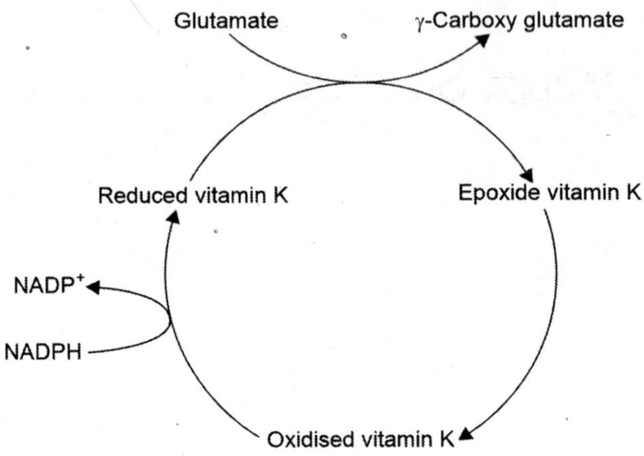

Vitamin K antagonist

Warfarin

Deficiency Manifestations

1. Hemorrhagic disease of newborn.
2. Bleeding from nose, skin, internal bleeding.
3. Prolonged prothrombin time.

CHAPTER

4

Water Soluble Vitamins

THIAMINE

Beriberi is due to the deficiency of vitamin B_1 or thiamine.

Sources of Thiamine

- Unpolished rice
- Whole wheat
- Yeast

RDA

1–1.5 mg/day

Functions of Thiamine

- Cofactor for enzymes of carbohydrate metabolism.
- Thiamine pyrophosphate (TPP) is the active form.

Deficiency Manifestations of Thiamine

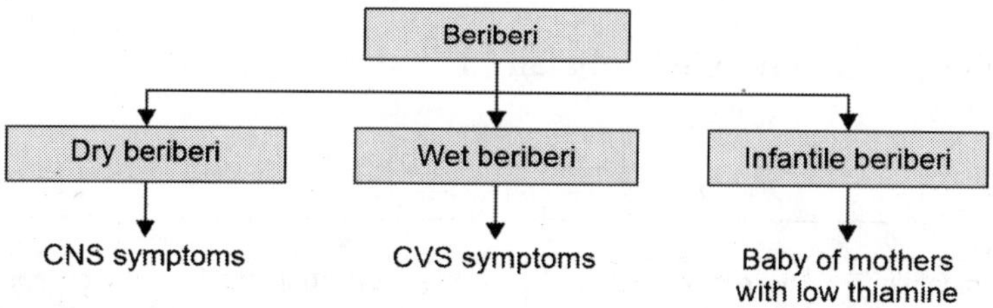

Laboratory Diagnosis

RBC transketolase activity.

NIACIN

Pellagra is due to the deficiency of niacin.

Sources of Niacin

- Unpolished rice
- Yeast
- Meat
- Whole wheat
- Liver
- Fish

60 mg of tryptophan provides 1 mg of niacin

RDA

20 mg/day.

Functions of Niacin

- Coenzymes NAD, NADP
- Carbohydrate metabolism
- Beta oxidation
- Fatty acid synthesis
- Cholesterol and steroid hormone synthesis.

Deficiency Manifestations of Niacin

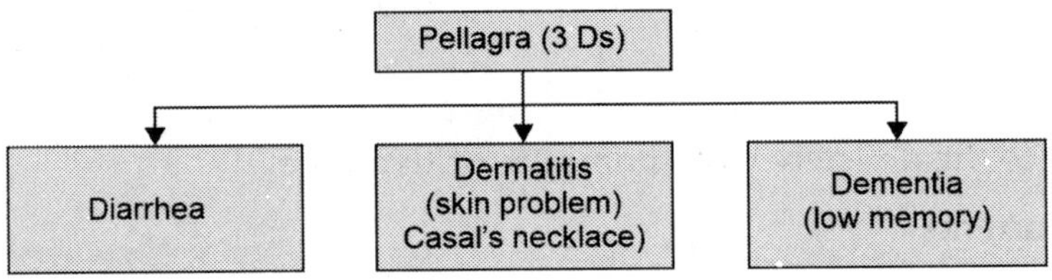

Causes of Pellagra

1. Maize, jowar diet.
2. Tuberculosis treatment (isoniazid).
3. Hartnup's disease.
4. Carcinoid syndrome.

Use of Niacin

It is used to decrease blood cholesterol and lipoprotein (a) levels.

VITAMIN B_{12}

It is a water-soluble vitamin called cobalamin.

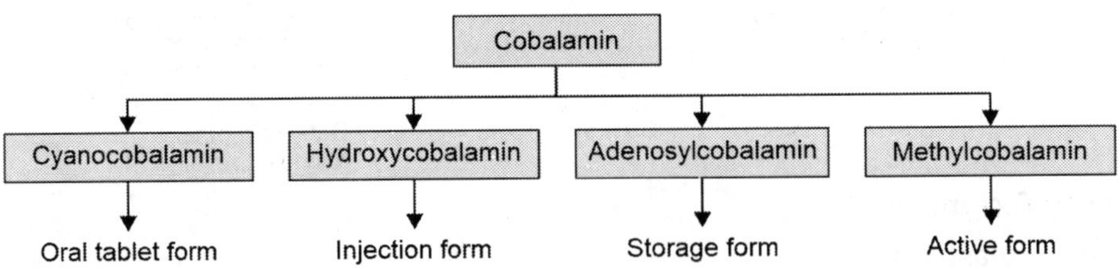

Sources

- Liver
- Curd
- Absent in vegetables

RDA

- **Adults:** 1–2 µg/day
- **Pregnancy:** 2 µg/day

Absorption

Small intestine → Terminal ileum (intrinsic factor + vitamin B_{12}).

Biochemical Functions

1. Fatty acid metabolism
2. Methylation reactions
3. Methionine metabolism.

Deficiency Manifestations

1. Fish tapeworm in the intestine causes vitamin B_{12} deficiency.
2. Megaloblastic anemia.
3. Subacute combined degeneration of the spinal cord.
4. Folate trap.

Laboratory Diagnosis

- Schilling's test.
- Serum vitamin B_{12} assay (ECLIA).

FOLIC ACID

It is a water-soluble vitamin

Sources

1. Green leafy vegetables
2. Yeast
3. Cereals
4. Pulses
5. Egg

RDA

- **Adults:** 200 μg/day
- **Pregnancy:** 400 μg/day

Absorption

Small intestine → Jejunum

Biochemical Functions

1. Coenzyme—THFA (tetrahydrofolic acid)—carries one carbon compounds.
2. Amino acid metabolism.
3. DNA, RNA, RBC synthesis.
4. Pregnancy.
5. Prevents cancer.

Deficiency Manifestations

1. Reduced DNA synthesis
2. Macrocytic anemia
3. Neural tube defects in fetus.

Laboratory Diagnosis

1. Increased blood homocysteine levels
2. FIGLU excretion test
3. Peripheral smear shows macrocytes, reticulocytosis.

VITAMIN C

- Vitamin C is a water-soluble vitamin
- Also known as ascorbic acid
- Can be synthesised by plants and animals.

Sources

1. Amla
2. Guava
3. Lime
4. Lemon
5. Green leafy vegetables.

RDA: 75 mg/day.

Biochemical Functions

1. Redox reactions
2. Collagen synthesis
3. Amino acid metabolism
4. Iron absorption
5. Methemoglobin reduction
6. Conversion of folic acid to tetra hydrofolic acid (THFA)
7. Steroid hormone synthesis
8. Antibodies production
9. Antioxidant
10. Prevents cataract formation.

Deficiency Manifestations

1. Scurvy
2. Bleeding in skin, nose and gums
3. Weak bones
4. Soft nails
5. Anemia.

Therapeutic Uses

1. Fractures
2. Wounds
3. COVID-19.

CHAPTER

5

Minerals

CALCIUM

Distribution

- 99% is seen in bone
- 1% in ECF.

Sources

Milk, egg, fish, cereals, vegetables.

RDA (Recommended Dietary Allowance)

Adult—1000 mg/day
Child—750 mg/day
Pregnancy and lactating women—1500 mg/day.

Absorption

Calcium is absorbed in the first and second part of the duodenum.

Factors Increasing Absorption

- Vitamin D
- Parathyroid hormone
- Acidity
- Amino acids—lysine, arginine.

Factors Decreasing Absorption

- Oxalates
- Phytates
- Phosphates
- Malabsorption syndrome.

Functions of Calcium

1. Enzyme activation, e.g. pancreatic lipase, clotting factors.
2. Muscle contraction—excitation contraction coupling.
3. Nerve conduction.

4. Hormone secretion, e.g. insulin, calcitonin.
5. Second messenger, e.g. GPCR and IP3 pathway.
6. Calcium decreases vascular permeability.
7. Blood coagulation. Calcium is factor IV.
8. Myocardial contractility.
9. Bone and teeth formation.
10. Calpains, cell motility, platelet aggregation.

Normal serum calcium level: 9 to 11 mg/dL

Estimation of Serum Calcium

- Arsenazo method.
- OCPC (O-cresolphthalein complex) method.
- ISE method (ion selective electrode).

Regulation of Blood Calcium Levels

Hormones	*Bone*	*Renal tubules*	*Intestine*
Vitamin D	1. Increase osteoblasts 2. Increase ALP 3. Bone mineralization	1. Increase calcium reabsorption 2. Increase phosphate reabsorption	1. Increase calcium absorption 2. Increase calbindin
Parathyroid hormone	1. Bone demineralization 2. Increase osteoclasts 3. Increase blood calcium	1. Increase calcium reabsorption 2. Increase phosphate excretion	Increase vitamin D activation
Calcitonin	1. Decrease bone resorption 2. Decrease osteoclasts 3. Decrease blood calcium 4. Increase osteoblasts	1. Decrease calcium reabsorption 2. Increase phosphate excretion	Inhibits calcium absorption

Hypercalcemia

Serum calcium >11 mg/dL

Causes

1. Hyperparathyroidism
2. Multiple myeloma
3. Bone metastasis

Hypocalcemia

Serum calcium <8.5 mg/dL

Causes

1. Vitamin D deficiency
2. Renal failure
3. Hypoparathyroidism

IRON

Iron is a trace element present in all cells.

Sources

1. Jaggery
2. Liver
3. Meat
4. Green leafy vegetables

RDA

Adults: 20 mg/day
Children: 20–30 mg/day
Pregnant women and mothers: 40 mg/day

Absorption of Iron

- Mucosal block theory of iron absorption
- Iron is absorbed in ferrous form in the duodenum and jejunum

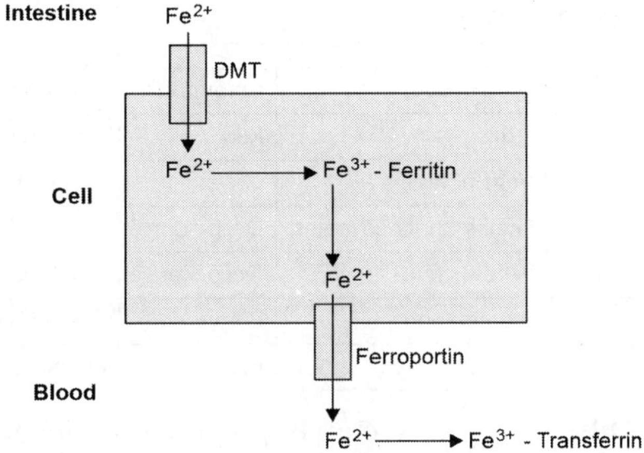

Absorption of Iron

Biochemical Functions

1. Hemoglobin—RBC synthesis, carry oxygen
2. Enzymes—cytochromes, catalase, peroxidase
3. ETC complex III

Deficiency Manifestation

Iron deficiency anemia—microcytic hypochromic anemia

Causes

1. Hookworm infection
2. Pregnancy
3. Chronic renal failure

Symptoms

1. Tiredness
2. Breathlessness
3. Excessive sleeping

Laboratory Diagnosis

1. Hemoglobin levels decreased
   - Normal level in males: 14–16 g/dL
   - Females: 12–14 g/dL
2. Serum iron levels decreased; Normal level: 100–150 µg/dL
3. Serum ferritin levels decreased; Normal level: 13–400 ng/ml
4. Serum transferrin levels increased; Normal level: 200–350 mg/dL
5. Total iron binding capacity (TIBC) increased; Normal level: 240–450 µg/dL
6. Peripheral blood smear: Microcytic hypochromic anemia

CHAPTER

6

Dietetics

FOOD GROUPS

S. No	*Food groups*	*Color code*	*Major nutrients*
1	Fruits	Red	Vitamin C, folate, fibre, potassium
2	Vegetables	Green	Vitamins A, C, E, fibres
3	Grains (enriched grains)	Deep orange	Vitamin B, folate, iron
4	Whole grains	Deep orange	Zinc, magnesium, fibre
5	Protein foods	Purple	Protein, vitamin E, vitamin B, iron
6	Dairy	Blue	Protein, calcium, phosphorus, magnesium, vitamin B_{12}

Oils: Not a food group. But supply essential nutrients like linoleic acid, α-linolenic acid, vitamin E.

FOOD GUIDES

1. Food guides are developed for use by the general public.
2. Intended to help people to select day-to-day food.
3. Helps meal planning.
4. Food guides group the foods based on their nutrient contents.

Examples of Commonly Used Food Guides

- Food guide pyramids.
- My plate.
- Choose your foods: Food lists for diabetes.

My Plate

1. This food icon was developed by the US Department of Agriculture.
2. It is an initiative to help consumers to make better food choices.
3. My plate translates dietary guidelines into action messages for consumers.
4. My plate plan website allows consumers to access a daily food plan based on their age, gender, body weight and level of physical activity.
5. It includes an appropriate amount of all five food groups which amounts to 2,000 calories.

Choose Your Foods: Food List for Diabetes

1. It was introduced by the American Diabetes Association.
2. Food list—group foods based on macronutrient content and equivalent energy value.
3. The food in each list can be freely interchanged and consumed without affecting the food value and calories because they are equal to one another in the indicated portions.
4. Food list is a useful dietary tool for control of carbohydrate intake in diabetes.

The food list arranges foods into three groups:

1. Carbohydrates—starch, fruits, milk.
2. Proteins—animal foods and plant-based proteins.
3. Fats—both animal and plant fats.

FOOD STANDARDS

1. In 1963, the World Health Assembly established the Food Standards Programme and the Codex Alimentarius Commission jointly with the Food and Agriculture Organisation (FAO) and WHO.
2. The World Food Safety Day is celebrated 7th of June every year with the theme "Food standards save lives".

Goals of Food Standards

1. Food standards are a way of ensuring safety and quality.
2. They define the maximum levels of additives, contaminants, residues of pesticides and veterinary drugs that can safely be consumed by all.
3. They are established following expert advice from food scientists, microbiologists, veterinarians, medical doctors and toxicologists.
4. Standards specify how the food should be measured, packaged and transported to keep it safe.
5. Food standards protect consumers by ensuring that the food they consume is safe.
6. Food standards help producers, processors and retailers to ensure food safety and to gain consumer confidence.

Codex Standards

1. The food standards can be developed by individual organizations, governments or by regional or intergovernmental standard-setting bodies.
2. One such international food safety and quality standard-setting body is the Codex Alimentarius Commission, or Codex for short.
3. Codex is the place where representatives of 188 member countries and 1 member organization (the European Union) work together to ensure food safety.
4. Codex standards are used as benchmarks by the World Trade Organization. If the food comes from abroad, it has to meet these standards.
5. Codex standards are considered as the heart of food safety.
6. For the past six decades since its establishment, each year the 'food code' grows– new standards are introduced and existing standards are revised as and when new data becomes available.

SECTION

VII

Molecular Biology, Immunology

CHAPTER

1

Structure of DNA

THE WATSON–CRICK MODEL

The Watson–Crick model describes the structure of DNA as a double helix, characterized by its right-handed spiral.

Key Features

- **Double helical structure:** DNA is composed of two intertwined strands forming a helical shape.
- **Backbone with phosphodiester bonds:** The backbone of DNA is formed by phosphodiester bonds linking the sugar-phosphate units of adjacent nucleotides.
- **Composition of nucleotide:** Each nucleotide consists of a base (adenine, thymine, guanine, or cytosine), a sugar, and a phosphate group.

Bases

- Adenine (A)
- Guanine (G)
- Thymine (T)
- Cytosine (C)

Chargaff's Rule

Chargaff's rule states that in DNA, the number of purine bases (adenine and guanine) equals the number of pyrimidine bases (thymine and cytosine).

$$A = T$$
$$G \equiv C$$

Number of purines = Number of pyrimidines

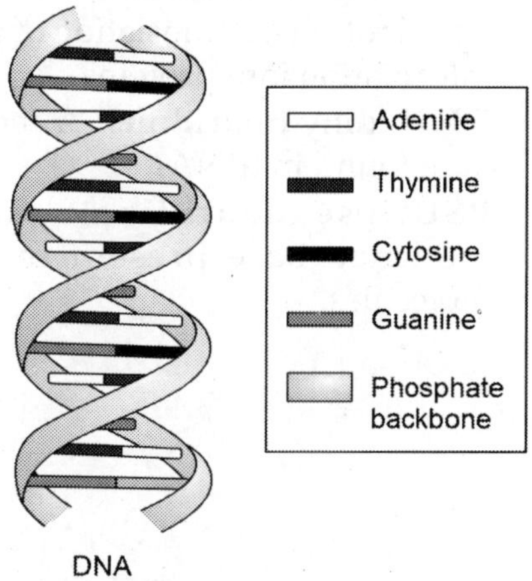

DNA

CHAPTER

2

RNA: Types and Functions

Ribonucleic acid (RNA), is crucial for various cellular processes. Unlike DNA, RNA is single-stranded.

TYPES OF RNA

1. mRNA (messenger RNA)
   – Carries genetic information from DNA.
2. rRNA (ribosomal RNA)
   – Essential for protein synthesis.
3. tRNA (transfer RNA)
   – Facilitates the transfer of amino acids.
4. snRNA (small nuclear RNA)
   – Involved in splicing processes.
5. miRNA (microRNA)
   – Regulates mRNA activities.

Structure of tRNA

- **Cloverleaf model:** The structure of tRNA is often depicted as a cloverleaf model.
- **Functions in translation:** tRNA plays a vital role in the translation of genetic information into proteins.
- **DHU (dihydrouridine):** A modified base found in tRNA.
- **PSU (pseudouridine):** Another modified base present in tRNA molecules.

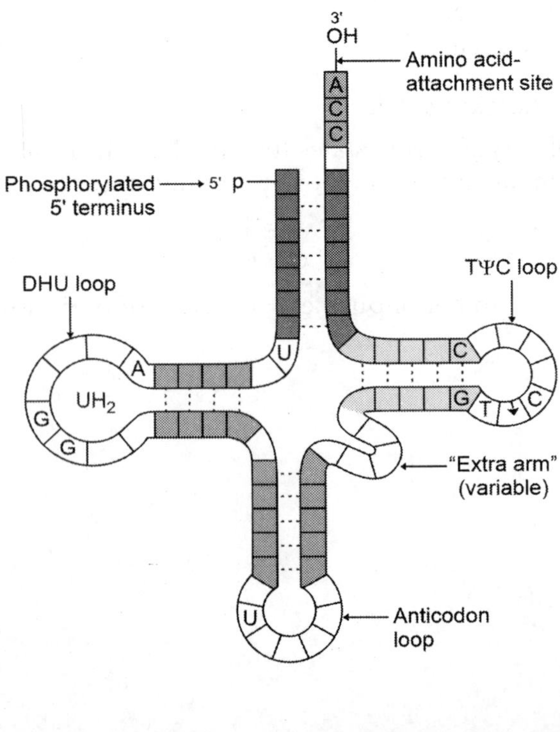

CHAPTER

3

Polymerase Chain Reaction (PCR)

Polymerase chain reaction (PCR) is a widely used technique for amplifying DNA or RNA sequences. It involves three main steps: Separation, priming, and extension.

Steps

1. **Separation**
   - DNA strands are separated
   - **Temperature:** 95°C for 15 seconds to 2 minutes
2. **Priming**
   - Primers are hybridized
   - **Temperature:** 50°C for 30 seconds to 2 minutes

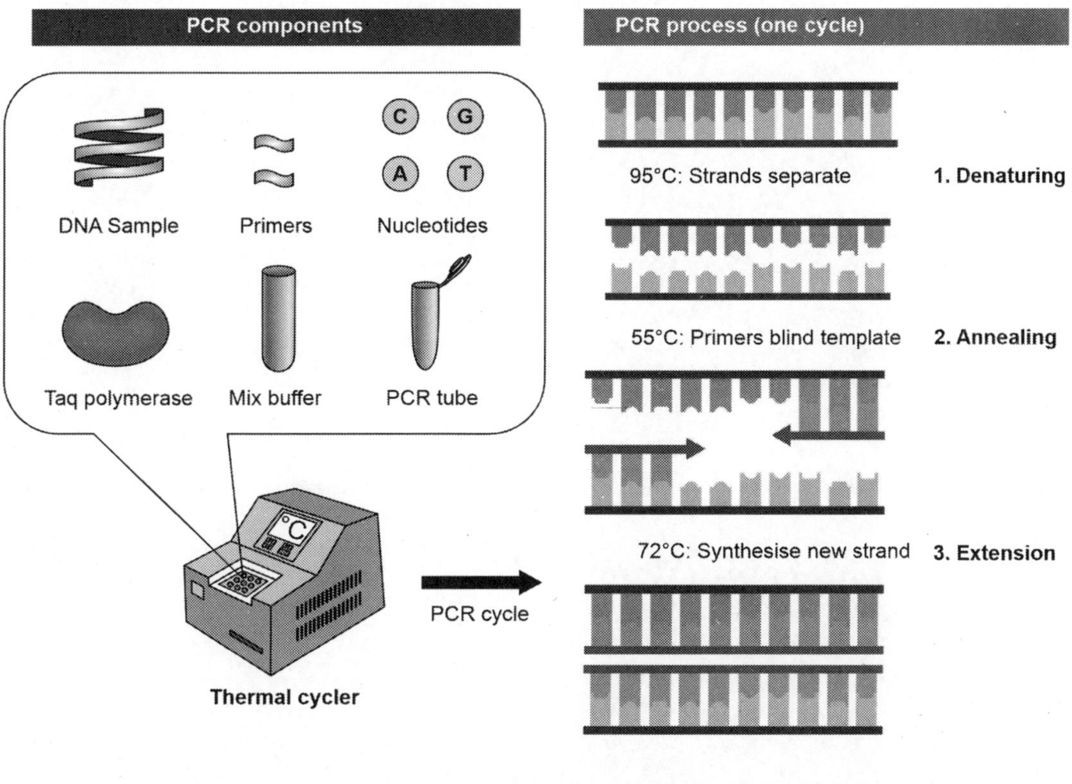

3. **Extension**
   - Extension is carried out by taq polymerase
   - **Temperature:** 72°C for 30 seconds
   - Cycle is typically repeated 20 times

Instrument: PCR is performed using a thermal cycler.

Applications of PCR

1. Testing for HIV, HCV, H1N1, and COVID
2. Tb testing using CBNAAT
3. Testing for cancer genes
4. RT-PCR for HBV viral load
5. DNA fingerprinting
6. Pre-natal diagnosis

CHAPTER

4

Blotting Techniques

PRINCIPLE

Blotting techniques rely on the principles of complementary base pairing and antigen-antibody specificity.

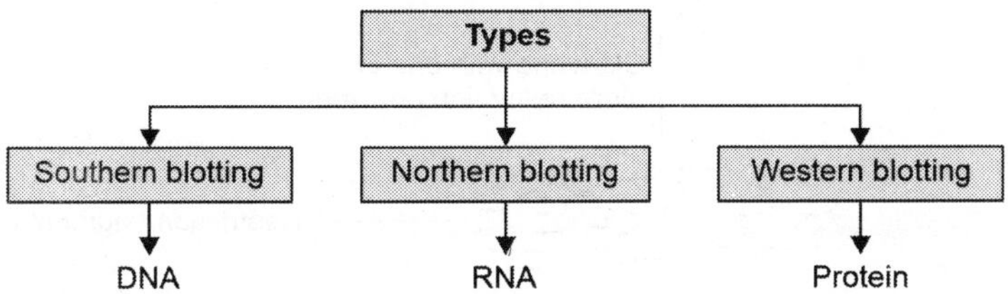

Southern Blot Technique

DNA fragments cut by restriction endonuclease

↓

DNA fragments separated by electrophoresis

↓

DNA fragments blotted on nitrocellulose membrane

↓

DNA probes added to the membrane

↓

Bands seen

Northern Blot Technique

RNA isolated from cell

↓

RNA separated by electrophoresis

↓

RNA blotted to membrane

↓

cDNA probes added

↓

RNA-DNA hybrid

↓

Detects gene expression

Western Blot Technique

Proteins isolated from tissue

↓

Proteins separated by electrophoresis

↓

Proteins blotted to nitrocellulose membrane

↓

Antibody probes are added

↓

Proteins are identified

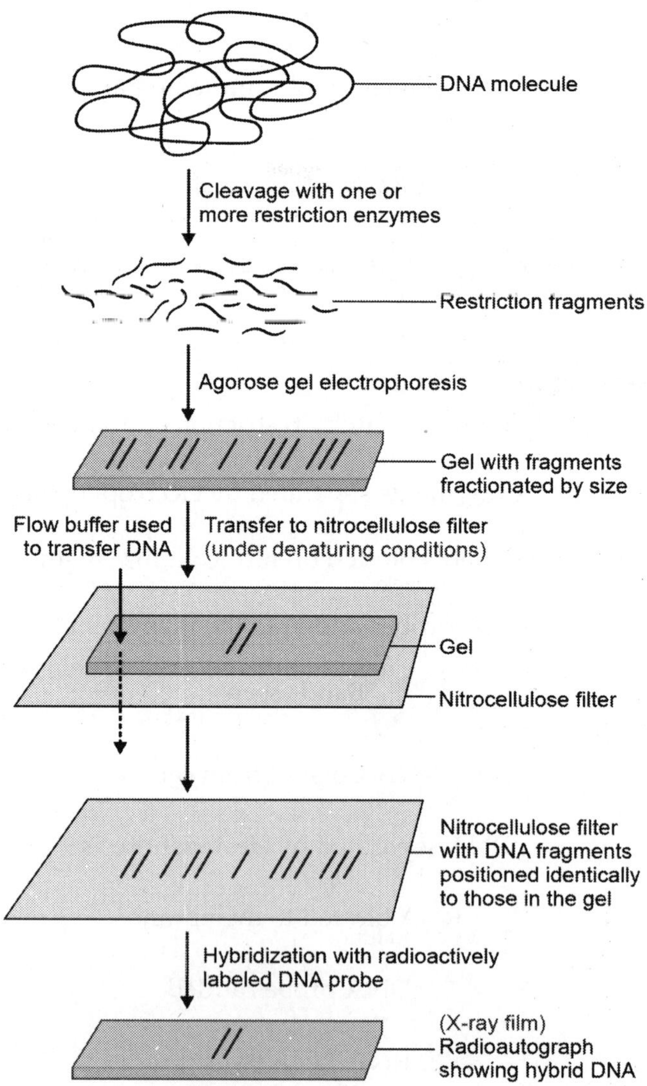

CHAPTER

5

Structure and Functions of Immunoglobulins

1. Immunoglobulins are antibodies that can bind to antigens
2. Antibodies are produced by B cells
3. Antibodies neutralize antigens

Type	*Heavy chain*	*Plasma concentration*	*Half-life*	*Functions*
IgA	α	13%	6 days	Present in secretions like mucous, saliva, milk, tears
IgD	δ	1%	3 days	B cell receptor
IgE	ε	0.002%	2 days	Allergic response, parasitic infestations
IgG	γ	80%	23 days	Major antibody, mediates secondary immune response, phagocytosis, crosses placenta
IgM	μ	6%	5 days	Mediates primary immune response, complement activation

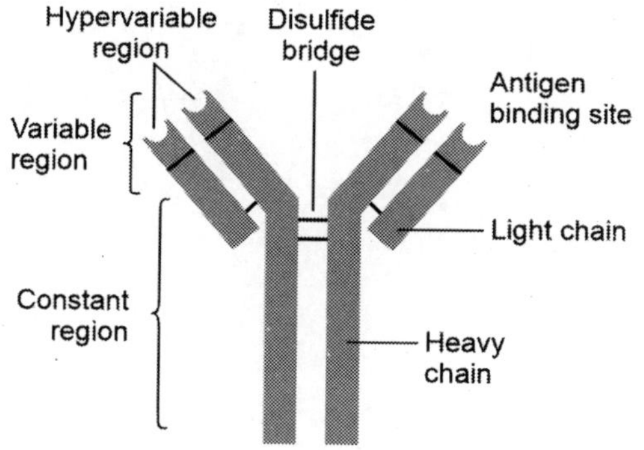

Structure and functions of immunoglobulins

Index